KAMA SUTRA

FOR BACK PAIN SUFFERERS

PROF GEORGE ZAFIROPOULOS

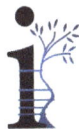

Guide to Intimacy for Chronic Back Pain Sufferers

and

People with Disabilities

IMPORTANT NOTICES / DISCLAIMERS

The depicted experience may not be considered as typical. Your background, education, experience, and work ethic may differ. This is used as an example and not a guarantee of success. Individuals do not track the typicality of its student's experiences. Your results may vary.

The contents of this training, such as text, graphics, images, and other material, are intended for informational and educational purposes and not for the purpose of rendering medical or mental health advice. The contents of this training are not intended to substitute for professional medical advice, diagnosis, and/or treatment. Please consult your medical professional before making changes to your diet, exercise routine, medical regimen, lifestyle, and/or mental health care.

This is not a medical consultation or medical advice. This is a guide to be followed, aiming to improve the quality of your life. You can keep all the material necessary for you and discard what is not working for you.

Stories shared during the sessions of the modules are true experiences of me personally, or of patients that have crossed paths with me during consultations many years ago. No personal details are shared within the course that can make them identifiable to anybody.

Author: George Zafiropoulos @2024

Title: Kama Sutra For Back Pain Sufferers

ISBN: 978-1-7384171-4-8

Category: Health/Self-help/Pain Management

Publisher: Breakfree Forever Publishing

REMEMBER:

Back pain is a symptom. Do not allow it to become a syndrome.

Intimacy is not a sexual act.

Intimacy is a mixture of love, respect, play,
communication and most of all, stimulation
of all senses.
Intimacy is sensuality mixed with sexuality.
Intimacy is pleasure.

Do not allow pain to rob you of your pleasure.

TABLE OF CONTENTS

INTRODUCTION

In this book, I am calling you to go through the possible ways that can be used so the effects of back pain, mainly chronic low back pain, could be reduced, leading to an improvement in the quality of life for all those suffering. Everybody who is a chronic low back pain sufferer can benefit from this book. Back pain has a huge impact on their well-being, and people's intimacy suffers. Professional and social lives are affected. Back pain can poison the way your loved ones feel about you, or vice versa, and create distances and barriers. Everyday activities are presented as difficult tasks, and relationships are frequently broken due to a lack of communication and loss of intimacy.

This book serves an educational purpose only and cannot substitute medical consultation, examination, and advice that someone could receive from their family doctor.

Back pain is a very common problem that affects millions of people worldwide. It is estimated that 9.4% of adults globally suffer from it. It is the second most common complaint that compels patients to visit their doctors, and among musculoskeletal conditions, it is the most prevalent. The effect on people in the productive age range is substantial. The productivity of people aged 45 to 65 years old is globally reduced by 20%; severe symptomatology can increase this to a 43% reduction in working hours. This leads to financial loss. On the other hand, it affects many other aspects of everyday life. It is reported that 81% of back pain sufferers experience problems with their sex life. Unfortunately, only a fraction of them discuss these issues with their doctors. Sex-related problems are considered taboo by many, leading them to avoid discussing them with anyone, including their partners.

One might wonder why one should concentrate on offering educational material to these individuals who do not even speak about their problems with their doctor. Some may suggest that this is not a topic to address and let the sufferers find their own solutions. However, why should this material be in the hands of every person suffering from back pain?

The answer is simple. These individuals, of all ages and genders, are in a state that prevents them from easily expressing their problems, leading to isolation from their environment and causing further emotional issues that can extend to their partners. As an empathetic fellow human being, I am here to help and explain to them that they should not feel forgotten and must feel secure and able to communicate about their feelings. People may question whether it is necessary to spend money and effort studying the problems of these individuals. Once again, the answer is straightforward. Human beings have built their existence in a social network. This network helps them to progress and thrive during their lives. It gives them the balance on which they build their future. This balance is based on many factors, but the most important is health. Health itself has its foundation in both physical and mental states, or better in physical and emotional wellbeing. Lack of contact and mainly lack of intimacy can create cracks in human relationships. Intimacy is fundamental to everybody, helping to keep loved partners close.

Back pain, though, may affect this feeling of closeness and frequently, by creating barriers, places the two people at a distance and makes them unhappy. Anxiety, fear, depression, and feelings of rejection may play a strong role and influence your environment. The repair of such traumatised relationships is crucial, and this is the reason you have to go through this book and learn the ways to manage both your physical and emotional state. In other words, your back pain, and your sex life.

But who am I and what makes me qualified to talk about back pain?

I studied Medicine. I specialised and became a Consultant Orthopaedic Surgeon. During my career, I have seen and treated a great number of people who had suffered from back pain, so I have a deep understanding of the condition, the implications, limitations, and effects on people's lives.

I have a total of over 43 years in Medicine, Science, and Experience on my side, and 39 of these years within Orthopaedic surgery. I observed the struggles couples were going through due to long chronic back pain issues and the difficulties they had while opening up about performance issues or fears during private moments. This is the reason I decided to write the present information.

I would be humbled, if you would allow me to share my experiences with you and assist your understanding of what low back pain is and how it affects us on many levels and systems of our body. The created material will guide us through different pathways, and step by step, we will find together the solution.

This is not a medical consultation, but it is an adventure through the cold corridors of science and the tumultuous ways of the mind. Both the body and mind suffer equally from this condition.

BACK PAIN AND PLEASURE

The reason I decided to share my experience with you became apparent when a patient of mine who was suffering from chronic low back pain during the consultation asked me:

> *"Doctor, can you please tell me how I can behave during intercourse? I enjoy being in the position where I straddle my husband, but afterwards, I suffer from a sore back for days. I would like to know how I can perform sex without experiencing this pain. Do I need to stop? I have asked people and tried to find solutions, but it seems that no one is able to answer my question."*

I have to say that I felt as if I was not qualified to answer such a question. I was surprised and tried to give a logical answer based on the science and mechanical function of the spine. That stimulated me, and I went on to study further to ensure that I can give correct advice.

A few weeks later, she came for a review. Smiling, she said:

> *"Doctor, you know you have solved my problem. I can say that it was a very long time since I had such pleasure and no pain afterwards. My friends may come and see you too. Thank you very much."*

She had spoken the truth. Since then, a number of patients of both genders came for a consultation for their back problems and inquired about ways to solve their intimate problems.

That episode and the subsequent patient visits enhanced my research, but I found out that there is not much information on the subject. This is the reason why I am here to assist you with my experience on how you can blend your pain with your pleasure.

For centuries, our ability to talk about our intimate relationships, particularly sexuality, has been considered tasteless, sinful, and shameful. This entire notion is based on cultural understandings developed over the last two millennia. Prior to this period, cultures in multiple territories or countries allowed people to freely express their feelings in a democratic way, without restrictions or taboos. They were able to admire nudity without shame and philosophise about the different emotions people had in an attempt to deeply research and explain their experiences. Unfortunately, changes in civil understanding caused these freedoms to be suffocated and become an "underground" dark discussion.

Someone could suggest that the book should only concentrate on women and not both genders. There is a reason to focus on the female population, and they may be right.

Firstly, women have been victimised for centuries as the "receiving," passive, non-dominant human beings who had no right to their own pleasure, beyond what they derived from sexual activities.

They were denied this, as they were not allowed to please themselves in the same way they could be pleased by eating chocolate or drinking a glass of nicely chilled water on a hot day or listening to their favourite music. They were considered, to use these vulgar, cruel, non-sensitive words, as lower-class individuals compared to male dominant desires, unable to express their satisfaction, as it was not permitted to them. This was the prevalent view, largely based on the anatomical differences between male and female bodies. You see, warriors had a lance ready to kill the animal they were hunting in the past, and the same explanation was allowed to dominate society, based on anatomical terms. Different cultures embraced this view for centuries.

The second factor is that since our existence on this planet, women have taken care of every aspect of common life.

Due to their caring nature and the ability to live a more organised life (male readers may disagree, but please reflect and think about the everyday activities and tasks your mothers, sisters, wives go through), they concentrate on the welfare of their families. This way, they have developed the common understanding that their pleasure must play second fiddle in comparison to everybody else.

This is the reason that although the book has a generic title including all back sufferers, in my opinion, emphasis must be given to women. In the end, they will, due to their nature, show empathy for their male partners and share their knowledge with them, as they always do.

The original *Kama Sutra*, although it demonstrates hundreds of different positions, will not be covered here. The focus will be on other aspects based on experimentation using all senses, such as sound, vision, taste, smell, and touch. It aims to educate everyone on how pleasure, respect, and love can be practiced. Pleasure is produced during intimate moments, but it does not only include coital activities. It teaches the use of all senses for greater pleasure and promotes the participation of both people involved in the discovery of such feelings. It is an educational tool indicating how to become a mate and not just participate in the act of mating.

In this book, you will be educated about the relationship between back pain and sexual activities and how they can be performed in a way that ensures your safety and manages your symptoms. You will learn how sex does not have to turn ecstasy into agony. You will hear how not to fear sex if you are a back pain sufferer, but you will also learn about how all other senses play a role in your satisfaction.

In my humble opinion, the book should be read by both genders, and I can further add that men, you need to know and educate yourselves about finding ways to support your partners, and women, you will truly find ways as it is in your nature to help your male counterparts.

But before I continue, I must make a declaration. I tend to write about men and women. This may be misunderstood as the book being focused solely on heterosexual couples. Even the illustrations may amplify this notion. Partnership has no gender and back pain is the same. It involves all and definitely both genders. Therefore, the book focuses on the vast majority of people. Within the pages, it may continue to use the terms "men" and "women" in writing, and I ask you to allow me to do so, but please understand that the word "man" refers to the penetrating partner and "woman" refers to the receiving partner.

This book is not about the actual act of sex, but about how you can experience pleasure, how to enjoy, and how to develop your sensuality despite the dark cloud of your back pain.

Before any details are presented, an analysis of the factors leading to pleasure will be discussed.

Pleasure, as mentioned before, is linked to all of our senses, including smell, touch, taste, sight, and hearing. Everyone, including each of you, is capable of experiencing and seeking pleasure through any single or all of these senses. If one of these five senses is lost, the others naturally become more prominent, allowing you to rely on the remaining senses. Sexual activity and the pleasure derived from it can be considered just like any other activity or exercise, such as jogging in the park or swimming in the sea, or even sitting on a breezy veranda on a nice summer afternoon listening to music or meditating on a yoga mat in the middle of your living room. This means that if you eliminate all other senses, sex becomes a limited activity. However, when all senses are engaged, this experience becomes filled with emotions, as the body and mind explore new horizons. These horizons encompass happiness, warmth, and immersion in a pleasurable space. But what effects does pleasure have on you? Pleasure serves as a means for humans to eliminate unhappiness and painful situations. This is why pleasure is linked and connected to back pain.

Any individual attempting to counter back pain creates defence mechanisms and strives to utilise whichever senses they can. The question then becomes: how will you accomplish this, and which senses will you activate?

Future chapters will provide a thorough explanation of the scientific mechanisms, shedding light on your reactions to back pain.

For now, let's concentrate on the ways in which you respond to the onset of back pain. People in your position often fall into a trap. They believe that by moving, the pain will return, and the symptoms will worsen. This fear dominates their thoughts, leaving them feeling uncertain, angry, and desperate.

When pain strikes as a reaction to this belief, the brain first reacts with panic. It orders immobilisation in this state of emergency. The condition known as kinesiophobia, or fear of motion, develops. The brain's command to remain immobile is driven by fear. You must combat this fear. It is well-known that movement and exercise can bring happiness, as the brain releases endorphins. Increasing your movement instils the confidence that motion is not harmful and helps address kinesiophobia. As your energy levels rise, you can gradually increase the complexity and frequency of your movements. Among the list of senses, motion represents touch, although it is more complex than that.

However, it is not just motion that has benefits. Stimulating our senses through music (hearing), being outdoors in nature (smell, sight, and hearing), or consuming specific foods (smell and taste) can also assist in managing and coping with back pain.

The same stimulation of senses and emotions can be experienced during sexual activities. However, it is important to discuss further the connection between back pain and sexuality, including reviewing any limitations in terms of positions that can be performed.

The ability to engage in sexual activity is essential for you, your loved ones, and especially your partner. If you avoid sex and create barriers, it can affect your partner emotionally, leading to feelings of guilt, anger, abandonment, rejection, fear, anxiety, and even depression. We know that back pain symptoms can create significant stress. In order to avoid this, it is crucial to communicate with your loved one and explain your limitations, emphasising that sexual activities can still take place, but adjustments to the usual routine might be necessary.

To be able to enjoy sex while experiencing pain, it is important to discover, understand, and become familiar with your own body, particularly under these new circumstances and any movement limitations it may have.

In order to do so, you need to determine the cause of your back pain and the extent of your spinal condition. You also need to identify the phase your pain is in, whether it is acute, acute on chronic, or chronic. This will determine the activities or positions that are suitable during intimate moments. Your doctor can provide you with this information.

It is crucial to rebuild the closeness with your partner and effectively communicate your needs. Share your limitations and concerns honestly, while also being open to your partner's support. Depending on the level of pain, you both need to be open to trying new things and let go of any taboos, shyness, or shame. Do not be one of those who avoid discussing these matters. It is important to have these discussions. Being intimate with your loved one is natural; follow your instincts. Fear, shame, avoidance, and guilt are emotions that can destroy relationships. Instead, focus on finding solutions and be positive, open-minded, and ready to enjoy the activity and stimulate all your senses, safely and with control.

Pythagoras, the Greek philosopher, once said, *"The person who is able to control themselves is free."*

On the other hand, another Greek philosopher, Epicurus, preached that *"All pleasure is easy to obtain."* This means that conversation, laughter, kissing, touching, hugging, or simply enjoying someone's company or dancing can easily provide you with pleasure.

But what do you need to know? In future chapters, you will learn about the pathology that leads to back pain. However, for now, let's focus on specific activities and movements that can simplify things. There are two fundamental movements to remember: spine bending backwards (extension) and spine bending forwards (flexion). These two motions are crucial in understanding pain creation based on the spinal condition. They will also help determine the comfortable positions to adopt during intimate activities.

So, how should you act? During the acute or acute-on-chronic phase, it is important to be gentle and adaptable, especially since routine positions may have been established during the chronic phase.

Additionally, you should find ways to support your back or your partner's back, if you are not the one experiencing the pain, during these activities.

In my humble opinion, both parties involved should read this book. It will shed light on the needs of each individual and promote mutual respect by fostering knowledge and understanding of one another.

Activity
Write down what symptoms stop you from feeling happy.

_____

_____

_____

_____

_____

_____

_____

_____

_____

INTIMACY DURING DIFFERENT PHASES OF BACK PAIN

In the following chapters, you will find possible activities or environments that you can explore to enhance your sensuality and sexuality, taking into consideration the phase of pain you may be experiencing. It's important to note that specific medications or simply being in pain can impact your desire for intimacy, due to changes in your hormonal balance.

Acute phase of Back Pain

During this time, the pain is very severe. Typically, the fear level is high, and you may not want to move at all. Your doctor may have prescribed a lot of painkillers, which might make you feel drowsy. There is a possibility that you may not want to be touched or may not be able to tolerate any activities. Usually, this applies to about 60% of sufferers, and women are generally more affected. Almost all women choose not to engage in any activity, with about 80% of them deciding not to participate in sexual activities.

Despite this, it may be possible for you to want to experiment with the matter, as you are part of this small percentage that is willing to be more "active." What do you have to do? How can you safely experience sexual pleasure?

The answer is hidden within the definition of sensuality or pleasure itself. As mentioned earlier, pleasure is a combination of all the senses. By creating the right environment, you can truly feel sexual or, better yet, sensual satisfaction. The key is to create an atmosphere that allows your imagination to transport you to the right pleasurable scene.

This entire scenario needs to be made possible with the help of your partner. Starting with romantic conversation, your sense of hearing can be stimulated. This type of communication, using gentle and kind words, can remind you of previous experiences and transport you to those particular moments your partner is describing. This way, you are reliving those moments. Additionally, your partner can give you a massage to stimulate the senses of touch and smell, using aromatic oils, perfumes, or even lighting scented candles. Candles stimulate both vision and smell. Playing with food, such as bites of fruit or chocolate, can stimulate the sense of taste. If music is added to all of this, the picture becomes even more complete. It is known that this type of play can stimulate both partners equally, as they are more connected due to the deep emotions and the shared fight against the fear, they both feel.

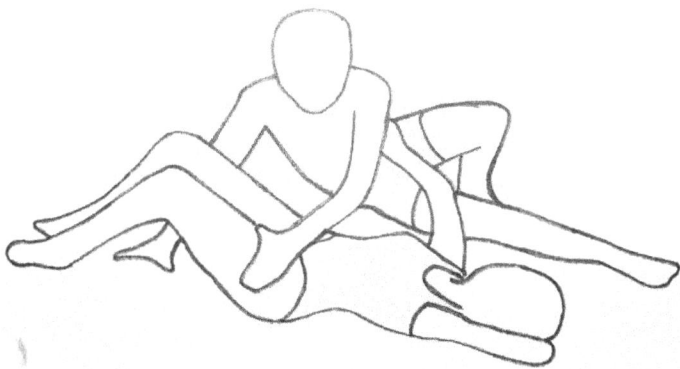

So, within this scenario, you can observe that all senses are giving you a general feeling of happiness. There is no movement, so pain is not elicited. The only thing you need is a very gentle, accommodating, cooperating, and loving partner. It is vital that both of you avoid impatience and take your time.

If you feel more adventurous, you could allow your companion to caress and kiss you, even in specific areas of your body. However, you must give strict instructions that if there is any pain, the entire play must stop immediately. Some may prefer to take painkillers before experimenting just to feel safe.

In the case of genital sex, it should be slow and gentle. People should respect and be cautious with their movements. Self-satisfaction could also be a solution in these cases, and in the case of two people participating, manual satisfaction could be acceptable.

In all cases, you, the person with back pain, should lie on your back, supporting your spine with pillows or small towels. Sometimes, depending on the cause of the pathology, you may need to place pillows under your knees to keep them slightly bent. You may also need to place pillows all around your body for added comfort. Most importantly, you should avoid sudden or forceful movements, and it is vital to remember that pleasure should be shared between partners. Neither of you should act selfishly. You are both a team.

If massage is chosen as part of the foreplay, the person with back pain may be temporarily placed in a prone position, and a gentle massage can be performed. Depending on the individual's gender, this gentle massage can transition into foreplay and may be extended based on the level of pain experienced.

Acute on Chronic Back Pain

What is the meaning of this term? It means that the person was suffering from chronic low back pain and is now experiencing a flare-up episode.

In these cases, a similar approach as mentioned above can be indicated. Usually, individuals are more familiar with their pain as they have experienced it before, so they are more willing to try different things. However, communication with your partner is essential. Creating a similar environment and engaging in foreplay would be necessary to help both parties relax and enjoy themselves. As mentioned earlier, the sufferer should be in a supported supine position.

Having knowledge of the pathology can help determine the position that someone should take or avoid. In the previous chapter, flexion or extension spinal positions were mentioned. Although a more detailed explanation will be provided later on, it should be noted that pathologies involving the posterior elements of the spine may tolerate extension positions better, while the opposite is true for pathologies present anteriorly or in cases of total degeneration, where flexion positions of the spine may work better.

Above all, the sufferer should have the lower back supported with either a pillow or towel, and both parties should be gentle.

Apart from self-satisfaction or oral sex, coital activity is also a possibility. In such cases, the following positions should be considered based on the sufferer's gender.

In the case of a male sufferer, the proposed position is as follows:

As mentioned in the previous paragraphs, it is much better for the person with back pain to be in a supine position with their back supported by a small pillow or rolled towel. In this case, the partner should straddle him, kneeling over him to facilitate penetration. There are two different positions for this to happen: the person on top could either face the person lying supine or have their back to him, facing his feet.

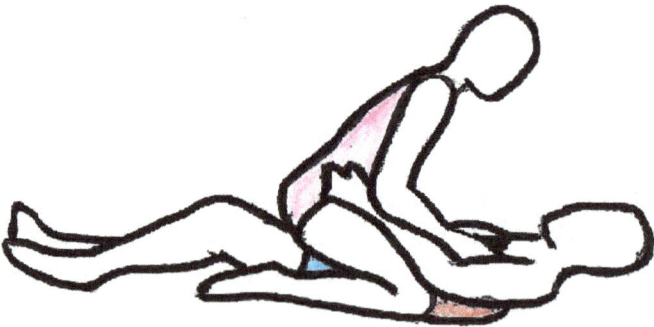

These positions are known by different names such as *"the reverse drop," "the deep press," "the seat of sport,"* or *"new leaf,"* depending on the variation and minor details. I won't go into detail about each one, but I want you to have a general idea and try to find a safe and pain-free way to enjoy pleasure in your life. Keep in mind that the entire act should be done gently, and if any movement causes pain, it should be stopped.

On the other hand, if the person experiencing back pain is a woman, the following practice should be followed.

The woman lies supine and is supported. The man positions himself between her legs. She should keep her legs with the knees flexed to avoid putting any stress on her sciatic nerve. He should make sure that none of his weight is placed on her, maintaining a position similar to that of preparing to do a press-up exercise. If the woman can tolerate some weight on her, a closer embrace can be performed. This position is commonly known as the "missionary" position, but in *Kama Sutra*, it is referred to as "the wide yawn" or "the flower in bloom." The act should be gentle, performed with care and respect.

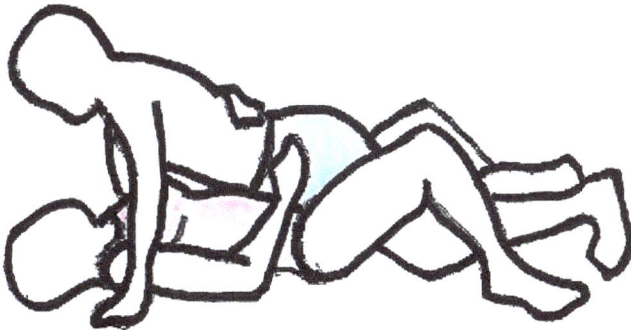

In the event that the woman can lie on her side, the man can approach her from behind to support her back and embrace her body. This should always be done gently, ensuring that his pelvis is positioned in a way that doesn't cause her any discomfort. This position is commonly referred to as *"spooning,"* but it can also be found under names such as *"parted waves," "halter of the princes,"* or *"playing the sitar."*

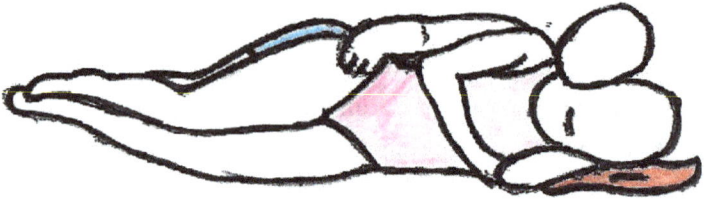

This, however, is a position that can be used even if the person experiencing back pain symptoms is a man. If that is the case, the posterior pelvic tilt is occurring in the woman's body.

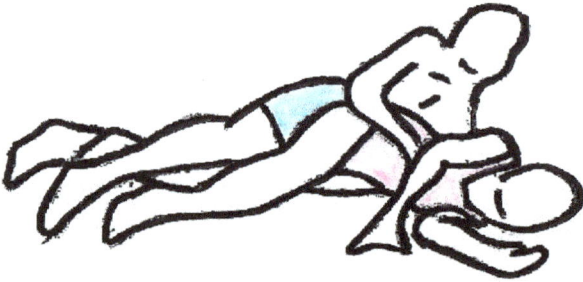

Finally, there is the possibility that they can both lie side by side but facing each other. This position can be applied when either of the two genders experiences back pain, making it a more or less universal position. In such cases, the pelvis of the non-sufferer is the one that can tilt forward, facilitating penetration.

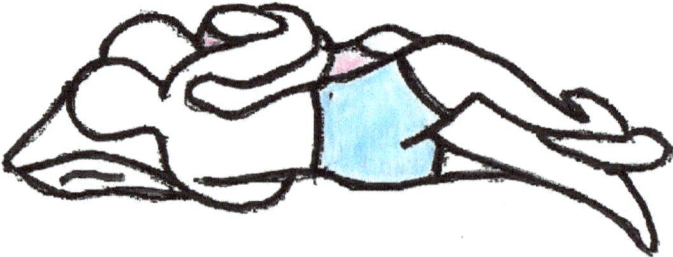

In all cases, patience, communication, and respect have to be the priority. You need to eliminate fear and anxiety, as these are very common and mainly because you are trying to avoid further pain and guilt in case the symptoms reignite.

Later on, you will find that in cases of acute pain, the sufferer has a lower libido due to hormonal levels. The most usual case is that the non-suffering partner is the person who initiates the act. However, this must not be against the wishes of the person who is suffering. Both partners have to be comfortable with the act, as even the non-sufferer may become anxious, worrying about the significant other's well-being. It is found that, in the end, after carefully planned and executed intercourse, the pain is getting better.

Chronic Low Back Pain

When the symptoms of back pain persist for more than three months, the term *"chronic low back pain"* is used.

In such cases, it can be said that sufferers already have some experience with positions they are familiar with and can perform safely.

Individuals with chronic low back pain have some mobility in the spine, but the range of motion is limited due to stiff ligaments, muscles, and joints. These limitations, along with the spine's pathology, can determine which positions are suitable and comfortable for them to perform without risking an acute-on-chronic phase. If the spine is stiff due to degenerative changes, most of the movement occurs at the hip and knee joints.

While spinal movements are multidirectional, when it comes to coital activities in the presence of pathological findings, the main motions usually involve extension and flexion. Rotational movements are very limited.

Later, we will discuss how the spine functions. For now, please remember that in the case of a disc prolapse or bulging, flexion should be avoided. The opposite is true for degenerative changes involving the facet joints (joints between the vertebrae). In such cases, extension should be avoided.

Dividing these two groups, you may observe those who prefer to stay in a lordotic position (leaning backwards, in extension) and those who find a kyphotic position (leaning forward or in flexion) more comfortable. Within these groups, it is important to further subdivide them according to gender. However, I want to emphasise that the terms "man" and "woman" are used figuratively to describe the penetrating partner and the receiving partner.

The reason for these groups is the need for different degrees of pelvic tilt depending on the position individuals have to adapt to, as well as the load they have to bear through their spines. It is evident that in the chronic low back pain groups, you, as a sufferer, need to be aware of your individual pathology and its findings in order to avoid worsening of symptoms. These findings would typically be provided by your doctor or can be found in your medical records.

• Lordosis – Lean Backwards – Extension

WOMAN

A

The most commonly used position is the *"missionary"* position, which is considered safer and can be used in the acute or subacute (acute on chronic) phases. Individuals are familiar with this position and feel more confident using it, especially if they have experimented with it in previous, more painful instances. Using a pillow, towel, or the arms of the partner to support the back can help women feel safe. It is advisable to flex the knees to avoid stretching the sciatic nerve.

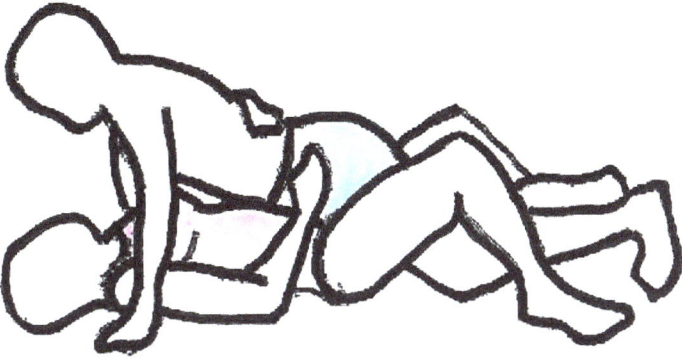

B

Close embrace of the two facing each other, with the woman wrapping her legs around the hips or waist of the man while he supports her back in a very close encounter. This position can be practiced on a bed while both are in a sitting position, or at the edge of the bed with the man sitting and the woman in a similar position as described before. This latter position may cause stress on the nerves if the woman carelessly keeps her legs straight. It is advised that her legs be wrapped around the man's body.

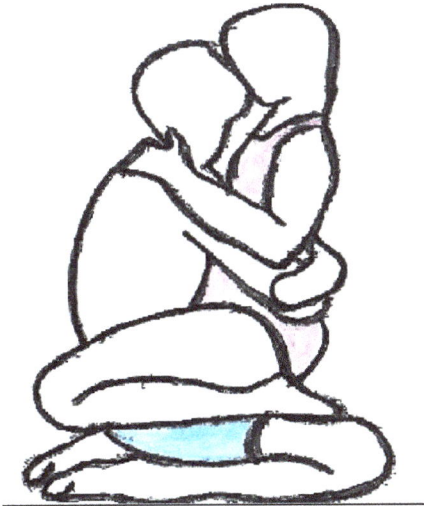

Finally, the same position can be achieved with the man sitting on a chair and the woman sitting on his lap, facing him.

Throughout all of these alternative positions, the man is holding the woman close and supporting her back with his arms. This latter position is called "the maiden's grandeur."

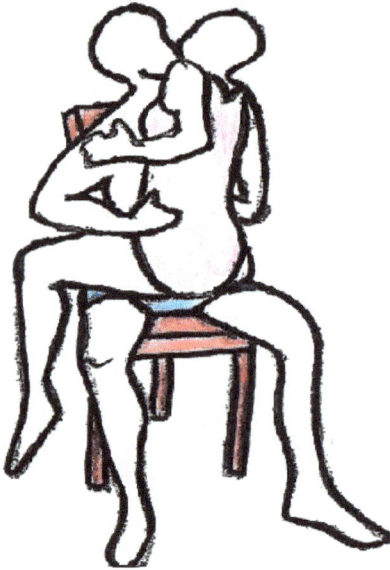

C

Almost in a similar way, but now the woman is facing the man and arching her spine backwards as she tilts her pelvis towards him (opposite position compared to the woman's body in the previously described position).

A potentially very comfortable position is when she sits on his lap while he sits on a chair. This position is called "sitting enthroned."

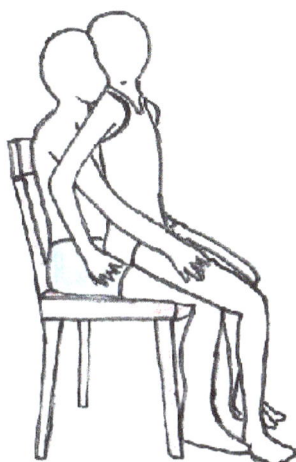

D

The woman is in a prone position with a possible pillow or other support under her chest to help her maintain the necessary extension her body needs. The man is approaching her from behind. This is the opposite of the *"missionary"* position.

The man is stabilising himself on his extended arms and is assuming the same position as in the press-up exercise. This position is called the *"Raised Flame."*

The woman's pelvis is slightly extended in order to accommodate the man.

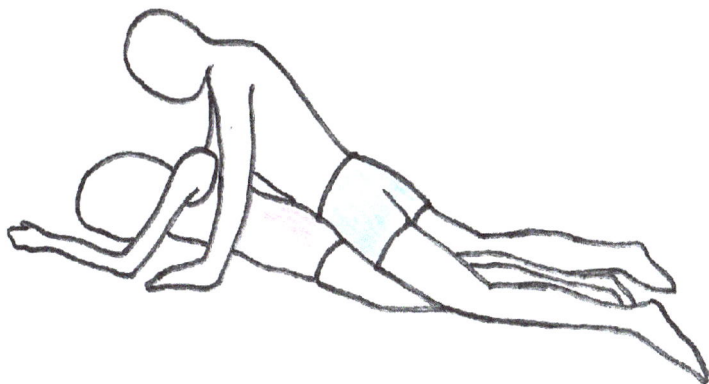

E

The woman is on her knees, bending forward and stabilising herself on her arms or on an object (such as the edge of a bed, a stool, an ottoman, or the seat of a chair). For her comfort and safety, to avoid any superficial abrasions, a pillow can be placed on the floor for her to kneel on. The man is kneeling behind her, while her pelvis is tilted towards him. This position offers her a lot of freedom, as she can adjust the extension of her back according to any discomfort she may experience. This position is commonly referred to as *"doggy style,"* but can also be called "the lioness supported" for a more elegant description.

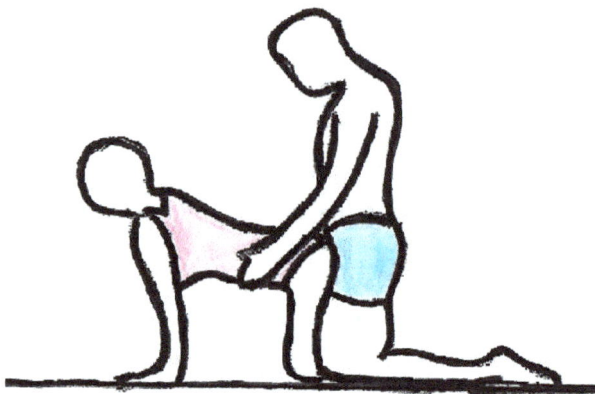

F

Similar to the above and to achieve the same result, both partners can remain standing. The woman is facing away from the man.

She keeps her legs slightly apart, and her spine is extended, tilting backwards.

By arching her spine backwards, she is able to control the extension based on her comfort.

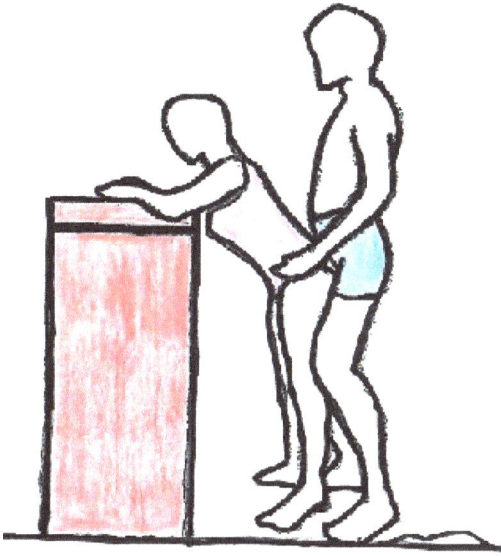

MAN

A

The *"missionary"* position helps the man maintain the extension of his back and adjust his posture according to his discomfort.

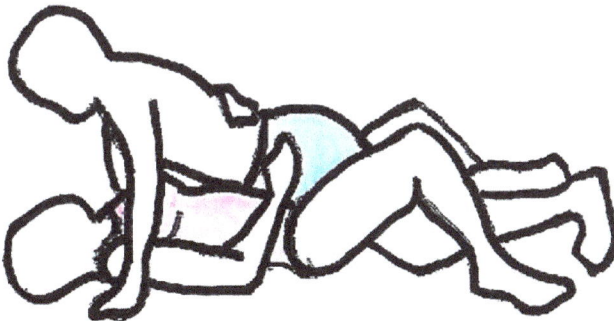

B.

The *"raised flame"* position gives him the exact freedom for better positioning of his spine.

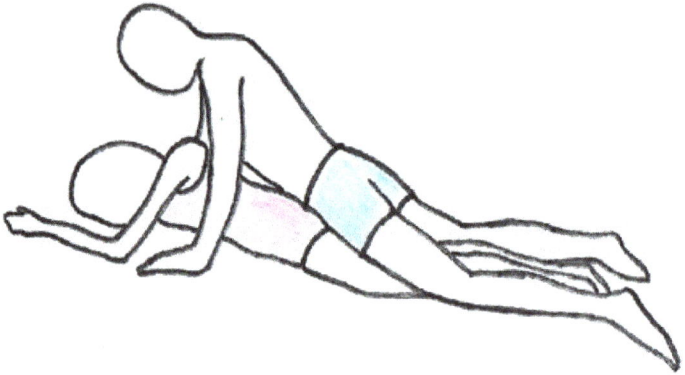

C

The *"doggy"* position again helps the man to control and adjust the extension of his spine.

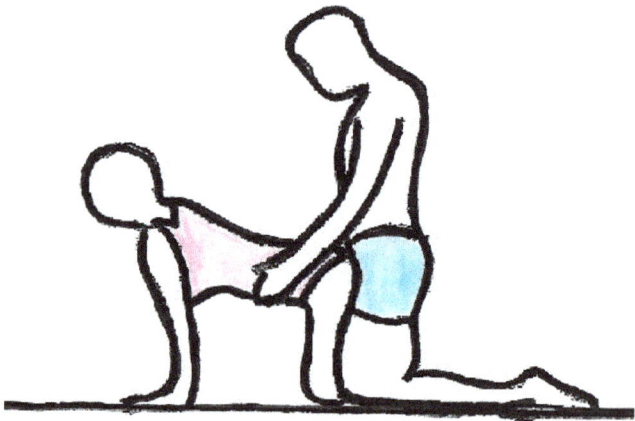

D

All the variations of him lying supine with a pillow under his back and having his partner straddled and sitting on him are positions that can be used and are familiar to him, as he used them in previous, more serious painful stages.

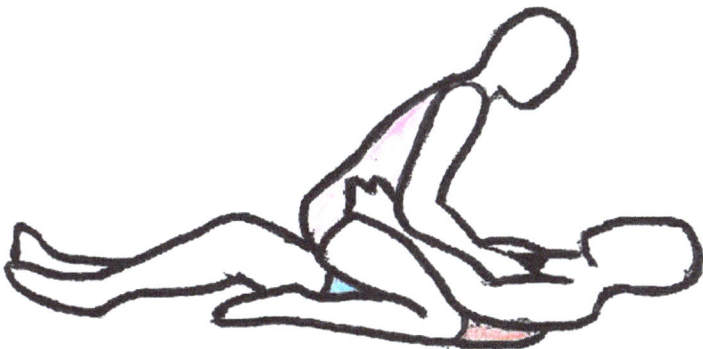

• Kyphosis – Lean Forwards – Flexion

WOMAN

A

The resurgence of the well-proven *"missionary"* position is possibly one of the golden standards.

A pillow or a towel could be placed under the small of the back if necessary to provide support. In this case, a flexed spine would work better. The woman's knees can be flexed further towards her chest. This flexion of the knees and legs can be easily adjusted in case of any discomfort. This position is commonly referred to as *"the rising lamb."*

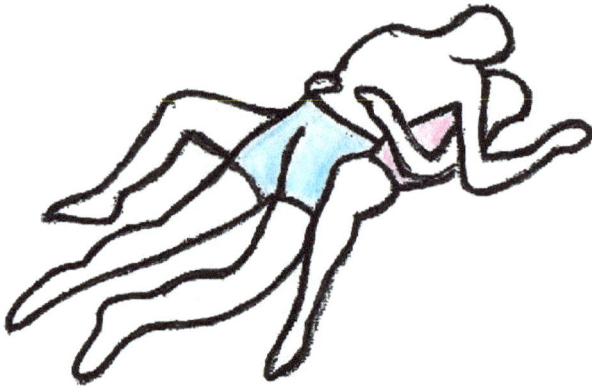

B.

The *"reverse drop,"* when the woman is straddled kneeling over the man facing away from him and bending her body toward his feet, is a position she can use to control the flexion of her spine and manage any potential symptoms in this way.

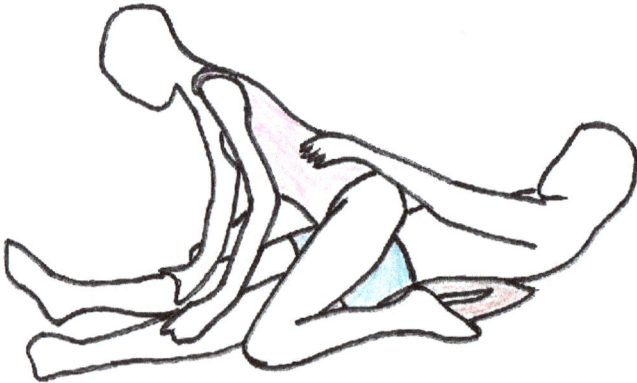

C

A variation of *"spooning"* is when her knees are bent over his body while she is in a supine position, and he is lying at her side at almost 90 degrees. This position is called *"the crossed branches"* and it keeps her spine in flexion. However, she will not be able to control or adjust her position, so she will need great cooperation from her partner. Usually, no back support is necessary.

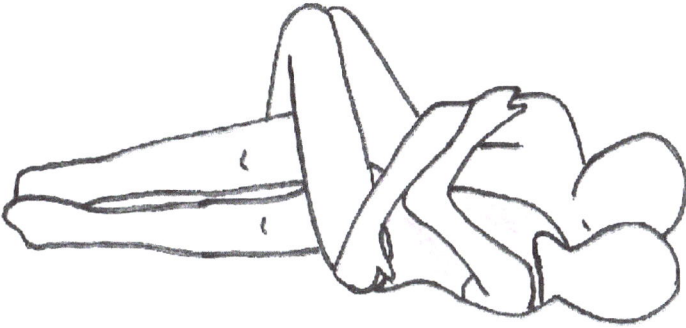

D

Variation of the *"doggy"* position with the stool or ottoman almost under her belly allows her body to flex more and at the same time be supported.

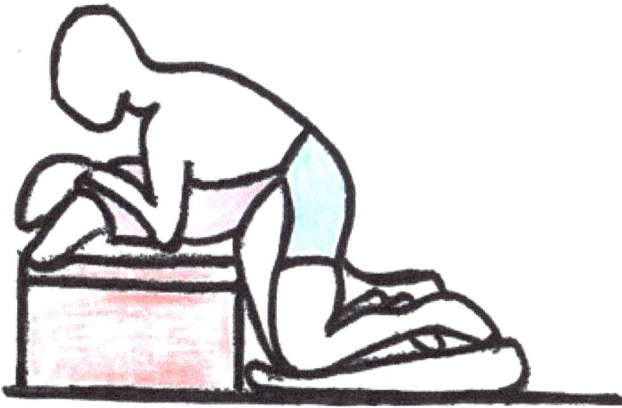

MAN

A

This is a variation of the *"missionary"* position. He is on his knees, and he has pulled the woman onto his lap with her pelvis over his thighs, holding and stabilising her pelvis on him. Her legs are wrapped around his body.

This way, he is leaning forward in an attempt to reach her, and he is forced to flex himself forward as he pulls her towards him. Although this position allows for flexion control, it also risks increased symptomatology if, under his excitement, he carelessly pulls her towards him by lifting her weight, which might stress his back.

B

Lying supine and having pillows under his back (dorsal area) while his partner straddles and kneels, sitting and facing him. His back can be in flexion while he holds her, almost *"hanging"* himself from her.

C

Sitting in bed, maintaining the position as described in the section on Lordosis for women (Position B), with the woman's legs wrapped around him.

These are possibly the most common and potentially safer positions for both genders that you might use as a back pain sufferer.

The "special" terminology for the different positions is borrowed from the book "Kama Sutra: A Position A Day" by Alicia Rihco, published by Penguin Random House in London in 2022.

Activity

Analyse your condition, identifying which body posture really worsens or eases your symptoms.

SCIENCE FIRST

I know that the majority of you want answers, as you want to quickly return to your daily activities, such as housework and taking care of your grandchildren. They are the pride and joy of every family and the future of our society. However, like everyone else, you want to alleviate your pain and replace it with pleasure.

Unfortunately, in this chapter, you will have to endure some scientific details. I will do my best to explain them as simply as possible.

So, let's begin with the science.

Back pain is a symptom of an initially unknown and unclear condition that affects our bodies. It extends from the shoulder blades to the lower back. To better understand the specific region we are talking about, doctors divide it into dorsal pain and low back pain. In this book, we will focus on low back pain and how it affects your intimate relationship with your partner. I want to emphasise that back pain is a symptom, but it should not deprive you of pleasure. If the back pain persists for three months from the initial onset, it is referred to as chronic low back pain.

There are 3 common classifications of back pain:

1. Axial, also known as mechanical, is present in a specific region.

2. Referred back pain is a dull pain radiating to the back from a different area. It can be global (generalised pain) or localised to a specific area.

3.   Radicular pain occurs when the pain starts in the back and radiates peripherally along the route of the irritated nerve, mainly the lower leg.

In the present, as already mentioned, we will be narrowly focused on chronic mechanical low back pain (localised in the lower part of the back) and its effect on your sex life.

I have to stress, though, that this material has only an educational purpose. It does not provide any specific medical opinion for specific conditions or individuals. It serves as a guideline for chronic low back pain for those people who do not present any red flags.

Red flags

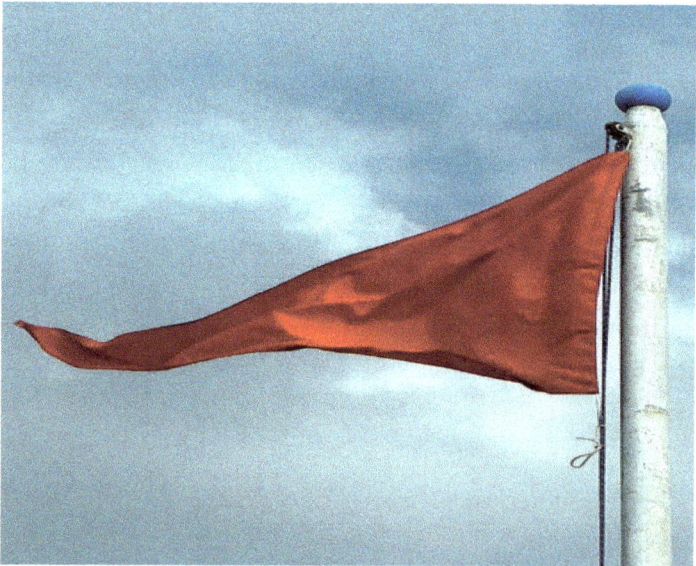

Red Flag: what is a red flag? It is the condition or symptom where if it is present to a person, this person has to visit their own doctor at their earliest convenience, because it could result in some unhappy consequences.

These are the most common red flags for a person presenting symptoms of back pain:

1. **Cauda equina syndrome.** In this condition there is 'saddle anaesthesia' present, meaning numbness or loss of sensation in the inner thighs, groins, gluteal region and perineum, loss of bladder or bowel control and weakness of the anal tone. This is an emergency.

2. **Spinal fracture.** This is the result of an injury. It could happen at any age, but for people above the age of 55, it could be presented as a sudden pain following a fall or minor injury on grounds of osteoporosis. It would be necessary to be investigated for the exclusion of the severity, pathology of the broken vertebra and possible further treatment would be necessary.

3. **Neoplastic deposits.** Usually these represent secondary deposits of a possibly already known primary malignancy. It is possible that the person may suffer from unexplained weight loss. Investigation, further opinion, and possible treatment may be the course of action.

4. **Infection.** Pain appearing suddenly following a recent or even longstanding significant generalised infection. There is the possibility of fever to accompany this pain. The condition has to be investigated and treated accordingly.

5. **Back pain associated with neurological symptoms.** Presentation of numbness or weakness of the legs, both or just the one. Further clinical evaluation would be necessary.

6. **Spinal stenosis.** Pain present in both legs after exercise, usually walking accompanied with mild numbness. The symptoms improve after the person either sits down, approximately the same time period as the time of walking or

is leaning forward and supports self against a steady object. Following this period of immobilisation, the patient is able to walk again without or with minimum discomfort until the next forced, by the symptoms, stop.

For all of the above, you need to see your doctor for further consultation, opinion, and treatment.

Who am I? As already mentioned, I am an Orthopaedic Surgeon and I have treated a lot of people with back pain throughout my career. This allows me to understand and empathise with how these people feel. I have been in practice for the last 43 years and I was trained by one of the best spinal surgeons. A great number of patients have come to me with back pain symptoms, and many have asked for my advice on improving their love life, as they fear that their partner has lost interest in them. Thanks to my extensive experience, I am able to explain and clarify matters for all. If you are one of those who suffer and fear for your relationship, I can assure you that I have done my research and found potential positions that can help you. All of these have been presented in previous chapters.

As I explained, achieving, and experiencing necessary pleasure is not merely about engaging in sexual intercourse. You need to know how to engage in it safely. You need to understand the scientific aspects and mechanics of your spinal movements. You need to know how to enhance and fully enjoy it, utilising all of your senses during this intimate experience.

I am here to offer my services to everyone, to share my experiences and to accompany all of you, step by step, on the journey that can lead to *"freedom."* Freedom from the intense, debilitating pain that demoralises us and brings us down into the depths.

But does freedom mean completely eliminating your symptoms from your life? The answer is NO.

According to Pythagoras, the Greek philosopher, *"The person who is able to control self is Free."*

In other words, freedom is the control of the symptoms; it is not the complete elimination. Finding ways to control and reduce the frequency and duration of suffering is a victory, and this is what everyone can call freedom.

You are in the depths of a dark valley, and you have to come out of it. You have to be "resurrected" by becoming free from all these troubles that have crossed your path and thrown you into the abyss.

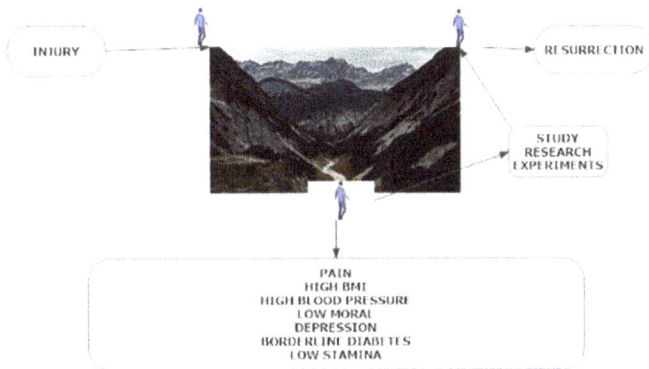

To help you, I started my own research and studied numerous papers and books for over 30 years. I delved into metabolism, endocrinology, chronic pain management, and the mechanics of the spine. After all of this, I successfully applied my findings and helped a large number of my patients.

I am now ready to discuss the steps and strategies that can help you overcome this burden.

I look forward to this challenge; I am ready to assist chronic low back pain sufferers in understanding their back pain and improving the quality of their lives. I want you to regain your activity and be able to take care of yourselves, enjoy your life with your significant other. I am here to help you eliminate mood swings, become happier, engage in activities with your loved partner, bring smiles back to your family, and do the things that back pain has prevented you from doing.

This is my purpose: to help you move forward, to help you escape the misery that back pain has forced upon you. I want to help you control your symptoms, experience pleasure again, and ultimately, achieve freedom.

To do this, you need to learn about back pain. Education on this subject is necessary, and I am here and prepared to help you understand it.

In the following chapters, there will be some more scientific information; unfortunately, it is necessary, but I will present it in a simple enough way. You will learn about the common causes and symptoms of back pain, but I will go deeper in explaining this. I will also discuss how back pain can affect people on a physical, mental, and social level, as well as the steps and strategies you can use to alleviate the symptoms and how to plan and implement these strategies.

I have already demonstrated positions that can help you find your way back to an active life with your most important person, your partner, by removing doubts, fear, and anxiety from your life. However, in addition to the practical aspects of these positions, you need to understand how your spine works and why your pain affects you. By acquiring this knowledge, you can experiment further and find your own solutions.

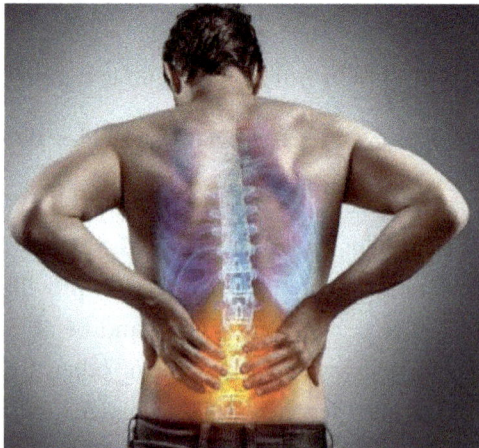

I must emphasise that this is not a medical consultation, and some strategies may not be suitable for you. Take what works best for you and discard the rest.

Activity

Please reflect and answer the following questions:

1. How long have you been suffering from back pain?

_____

_____

2. How was this back pain presented to you?

_____

_____

3. What have you done to try to improve it?

_____

_____

4. What is your current state?

_____

_____

5. What limitations do you have?

_____

_____

WHAT IS BACK PAIN?

We all know what back pain is, as we have experienced it, but do we really understand it?

Physically, back pain is present in our back, most often in the small of the back. It can spread to both buttocks, giving the feeling of a heavy load or sometimes a dull or sharp squeeze in the area, resembling a vice. Other times, it presents itself like a broad belt starting from the centre of our lower back and spreading to our sides, involving our core from the ribs down.

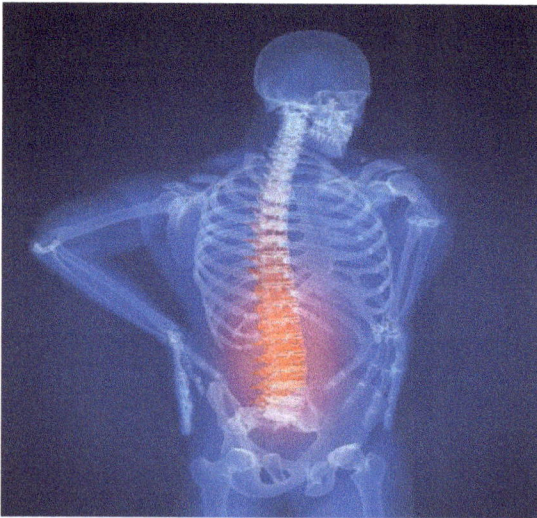

There are times when it appears as a sharp stabbing feeling that can take your breath away, and you look like a surprised person who does not understand where this lightning bolt came from. But other times, it can be deceiving and represented as a "sweet" stiffness that stops any movement of the body. It feels like a tooth of a gear came out of place from the existing "gears" of your body machine, and you start rotating, bending, and twisting in your attempt to put it back in place so that you can continue the motion you initially started.

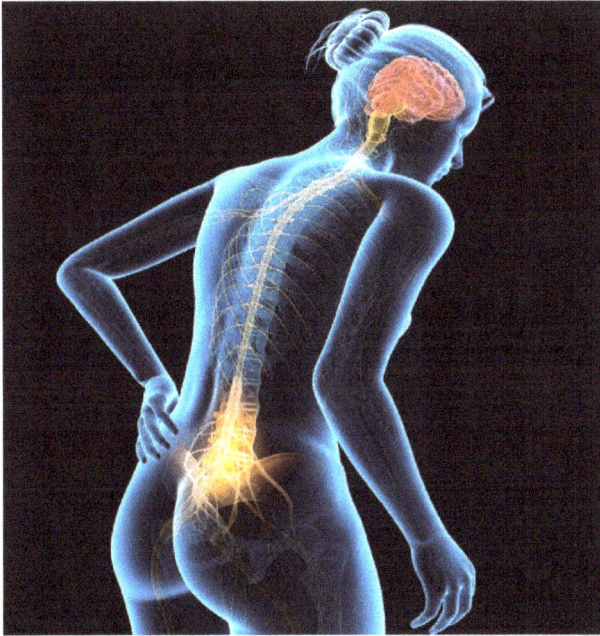

In addition to all of this, there are times when the pain spreads well beyond the buttocks toward the sides of the hips or down to the leg or both legs. Even this can vary. It can be a nagging or sharp pain with the presence of numbness in part of the leg, or it can spread to both legs. It can be there constantly, or it can only arise after we have walked for some time. This latter symptomatology can force us to stop and sit on a bench for almost the same amount of time that we spent walking, so that we can enjoy the surroundings or the sunset. Alternatively, it can make us bend and lean forward onto the nearby existing railing of the neighbour's fence and try to make friends with the dog that is roaming in the front garden. There are, however, these scary moments when the pain and numbness are so severe that you may lose control of your bodily functions and end up wet and dirty, not knowing how all of this happened. This fills your heart with fear. The main symptomatology described is that of spinal stenosis, although the latter symptoms present neurological dysfunction due to pressure on the spinal cord. Within the paragraphs above, some of the described symptoms may also be present when a Red Flag exists.

These are the majority of the most frequent presentations of back pain that people suffer from. These symptoms are described as a representation of a "monster" that hits them, torturing them and making their life miserable. But do not forget that back pain is a symptom, not a diagnosis.

As explained, this book focuses on mechanical back pain; we ignore any pain with neurological symptoms.

The inability to move freely and get out of bed in the morning could be the main problem for months. In the initial stages, you may need assistance from your significant other to be pulled out of bed every morning. Morale becomes very low. The family could be stressed to the maximum. Participation at the dinner table may be limited. Social and intimate life can become restricted and stressful. This could lead you to withdraw, stop communicating, and retreat into yourself like a tortoise in its shell.

The whole situation has a great effect on the family, and as communication is lost, the fear of rejection is *"floating in the air"* for both you and your partner. Intimacy is lacking, and the bonds holding your family together may start to erode and weaken.

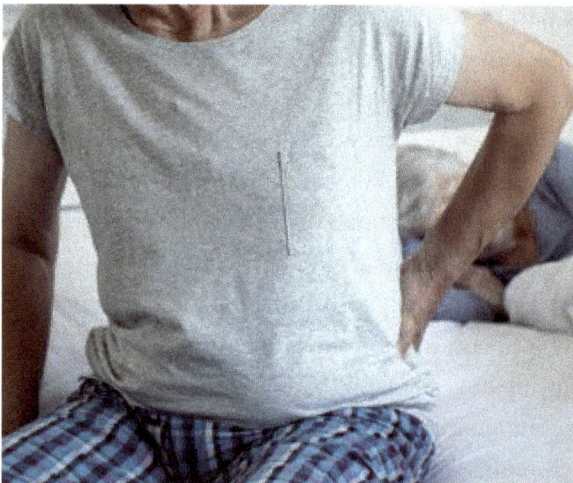

What was the mechanism that forced you to act like that?

In the following paragraphs, the effects of chronic back pain on your body and the mechanical function of the spine will be presented.

The primary physical symptom experienced by someone suffering from low back pain in the initial stages is a restriction of mobility. This affects the everyday activities that person can perform, both at home and at work. At the same time, emotions flood your brain and have a greater impact on you. This is the time when you need to understand what is happening, seek guidance, and educate yourself about back pain, how to modify your activities, and how to continue with your physical activities.

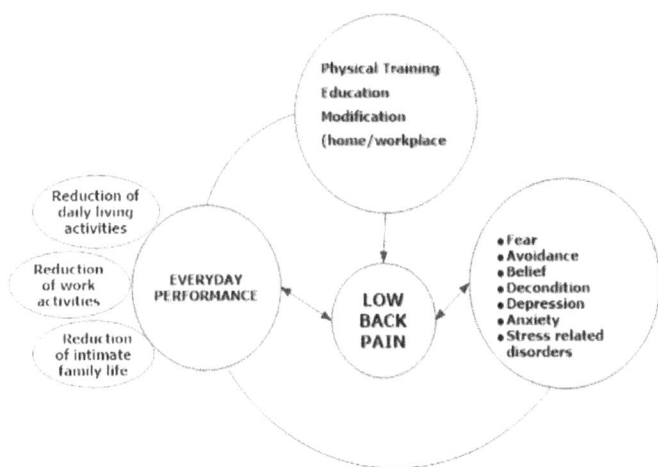

From the diagram above, it is obvious that mechanical low back pain in the initial stages not only affects daily activities, but also has a significant impact on another aspect of your life - your emotions. It can create fear and various other severe emotional symptoms.

Initially, it was believed that physical education and training were not influenced by the emotional sphere. However, this is not entirely true. They are indeed affected and can, in turn, affect emotions.

So, what mechanisms does the body go through?

Just the mention of *"back pain"* causes your brain to go into high alert. Fear fills your mind, and your breathing quickens as adrenaline and cortisol rush uncontrollably through your veins, urging you to run and escape from the grip of a monster. But as you soon realise, you can't escape. Your back is not letting go; it has bound you with chains and keeps you captive.

It is at this moment that your mental reaction starts causing more problems. It all begins with the reaction of your primitive brain, which is part of your brain. It kicks in, and the mechanisms of escape influence your developed brain. These mechanisms trigger more fear and anxiety, clouding your mind with emotions, and setting off a panic reaction - like a fish out of water. Your mind screams with despair, preventing any rational thoughts as your emotions flood your entire being. You struggle to understand how and why this is happening to you.

One thing, however, is clear. With physiotherapy, movement, education, and some modifications in your daily mobility, there is a strong possibility that the condition can be controlled in these early stages. This approach can help alleviate the emotional burden, as movement gives you confidence and confidence bring happiness. Thus, it is evident from the diagram below that movement can indeed impact your emotions.

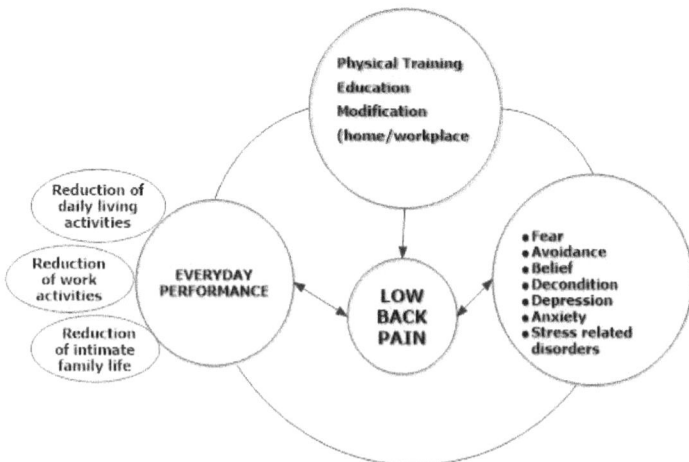

On the other hand, when back pain is present for more than three (3) months, it is considered chronic and the reaction is a bit different.

The initial cause of the pain could be the same or different than that of the acute phase, but there is a greater influence on your mental status to the extent that even your social life is affected. Intimate moments are avoided due to stress, fear, anxiety, and the belief that all activities will trigger a relapse of symptoms. As a result, your significant other also suffers. This is when the quality of your life is affected.

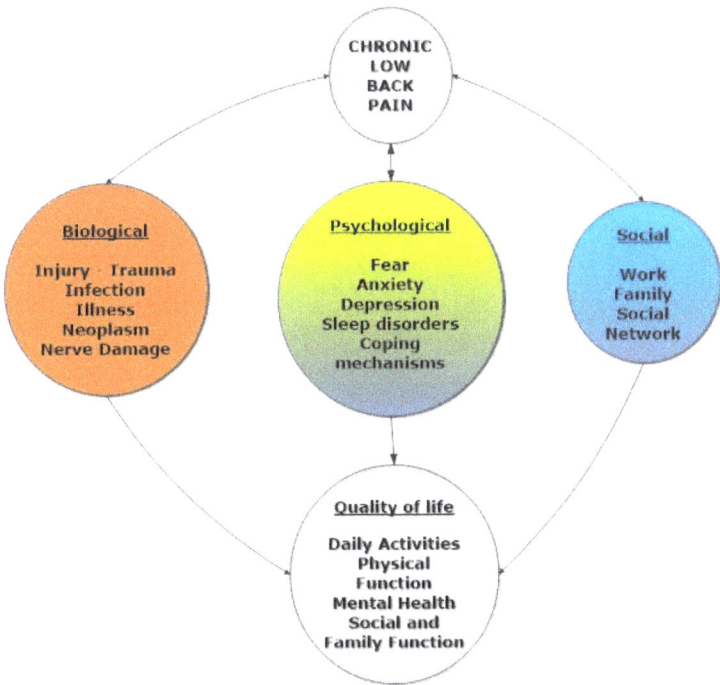

From this diagram, someone can observe that chronic low back pain has an indirect effect on the quality of your life. By affecting your psychology and social life, it places a heavy burden on your life. The physical, as well as the psychosocial issues, can fuel the back pain, creating a vicious circle. There is also a direct influence between these three aspects. You live a life filled with frustration, disappointment, and despair. All of this is better illustrated in the diagram below.

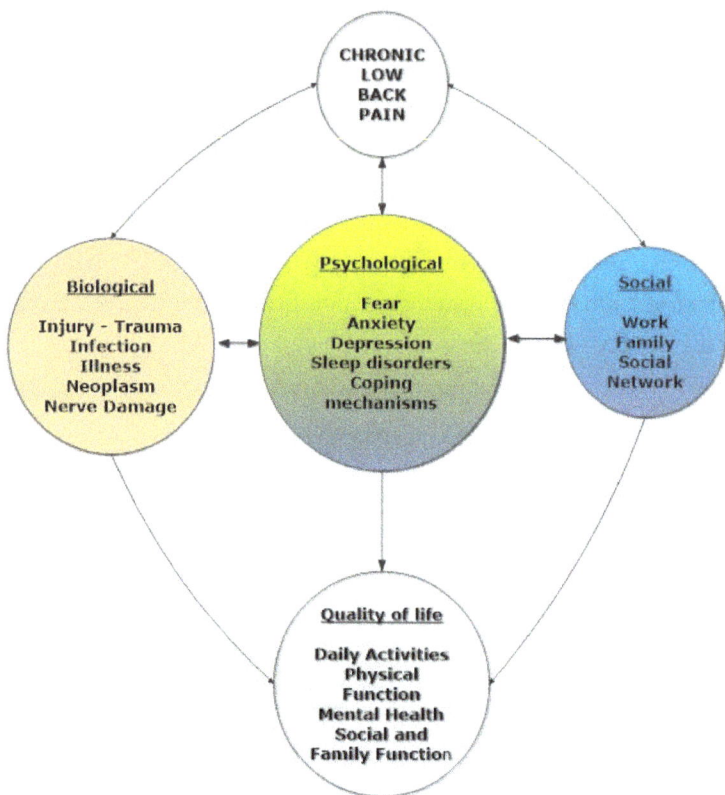

CHRONIC LOW BACK PAIN

Biological

Injury - Trauma
Infection
Illness
Neoplasm
Nerve Damage

Psychological

Fear
Anxiety
Depression
Sleep disorders
Coping
mechanisms

Social

Work
Family
Social
Network

Quality of life

Daily Activities
Physical
Function
Mental Health
Social and
Family Function

There is, however, a theoretical question.

Is back pain truly your enemy, as you may think, or is it your friend?

Do not forget that back pain is a symptom, not a diagnosis.

You may have had the injury years ago and the symptoms may have settled, but now you are experiencing pain again. Why did it present now and not two or three years ago? What is the reason?

Do you need to fight it or learn to understand it and be able to live with it?

You all know the story of Dennis, nicknamed the *"Menace,"* who initially annoyed the elderly man living next to his house with "inappropriate activities," but in the end, he became a valuable friend. Can you consider back pain a friend, though? This is a matter of opinion.

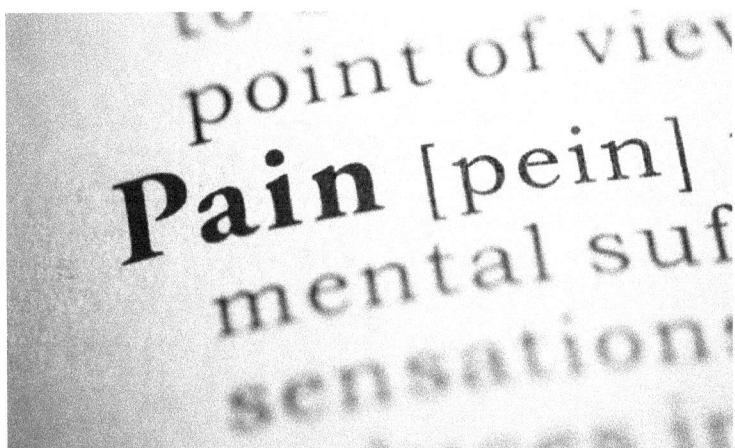

It depends on the perspective from which someone sees it. If you view it as an enemy and nothing else, then you have to fight it. You know that fights can cause injuries to both parties. On the other hand, if it is a friend, why is it causing these horrible symptoms and why are you suffering? There is, however, the possibility that it is trying to protect you from movements that can cause more damage to your body. You must not forget that most of the time, mechanical back pain is linked to an injury that occurred in the past, either acutely or through repetitive stressful actions. In the initial stages, you brace yourselves and try to heal the underlying cause. Back pain seems to be a defensive mechanism of your body. Upon further analysis, back pain is a symptom and not the condition itself. The problem is that you take this symptom and reinforce it in your brain, which leads to a cycle of bracing, muscle spasms, and secondary functional pains. This way, you are driving yourselves towards chronic low back pain and ongoing suffering. You are turning a symptom into a syndrome. Additionally, you are allowing this condition to rob you of pleasure in your life.

What causes back pain? Some of the causes of back pain, according to literature, are:

Biological	Occupational activities	Mental health issues	Non-direct spinal condition
Injury/strain resulting to muscle, ligament, disc, or bone tissue damage	Bad posture/ positioning	Sleeping disorders	Smoking
Degeneration of the tissues	Bad physical exercise	Depression	Pregnancy
Structural problems / Abnormal curvatures	Poor physical fitness	Anxiety	Shingles
High BMI (Body Mass Index)	Sedentary lifestyle		Kidney disease
Osteoporosis			Menstrual circle
Age			

In the diagram below, you can observe that spinal loading is higher when you are sitting than when you are standing upright.

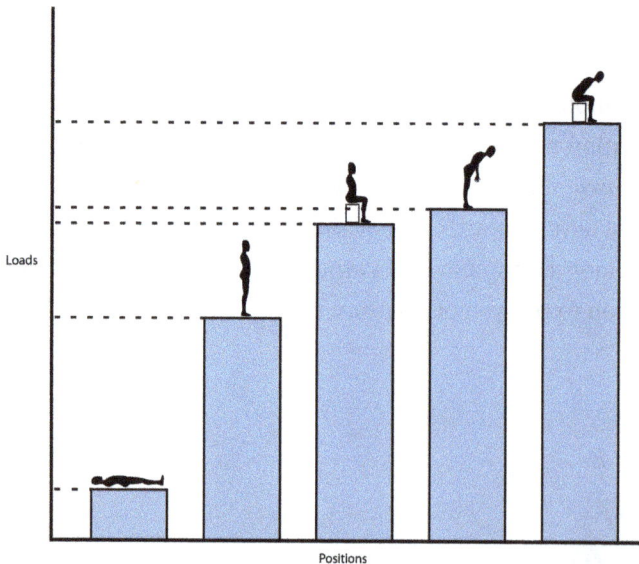

So, my friends, just sit back, calm down and enjoy the ride on your journey to learn how to live with your back pain as a friend and not as an enemy.

We need to learn:

1. How the spine works.

2. What can cause the pain to increase.

3. How we can address approach this issue that has come to our attention.

SPINAL MECHANISM

Spine and the neural system (including the central nerves and brain) are the first structures that are formed in our embryonic life. When fully developed, the spine is composed of a series of *"cylindrical"* bones called vertebrae, which are linked together like a bicycle chain. Behind these cylindrical bones, there are some arches that, when stacked on top of each other, create a tube known as the spinal canal. Within this canal, for most of the length of the spine, runs the spinal cord, which consists of nerve tissue and is a continuation of our brain. At the lower levels of this spinal tube and at the end of the cord, there are only nerve roots inside the canal. Due to their appearance, we refer to them as the cauda equina, which is Latin for *"horse tail"* because that is what they resemble. Along the spinal cord, we have nerve roots that exit the canal at each level and, once they exit, they connect with each other at different levels to form the peripheral nerves that extend throughout the body.

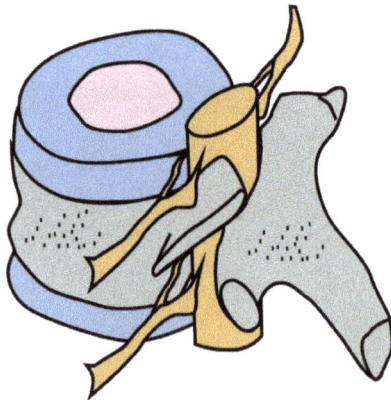

The spine, if we see it from the front, is straight for its entire length. However, if we see it from the side, it is curved. There are four different curvatures, two curving forward and two curving backward. The neck and lower back part lean backwards, while the dorsal and sacral area lean forwards. The forward curves are called kyphotic, and the backward curves are called lordotic. These names may help you understand the terminology in case you read a report from an investigation you have conducted.

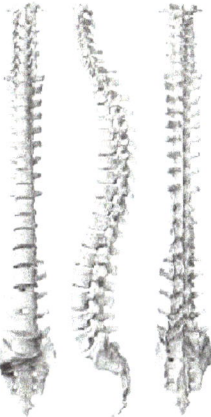

 The vertebrae are linked together with joints, which are part of the arch called facet joints, as well as ligaments that run in the front, back, and sides of the vertebrae. The joints are covered by a capsule and their own ligaments.

Between each level of vertebrae, we have another structure called the intervertebral disc. Discs are mainly composed of two parts: an elastic but firm ring called the annulus, and a central jelly-like substance called the nucleus. The nucleus is under tension within the entire structure.

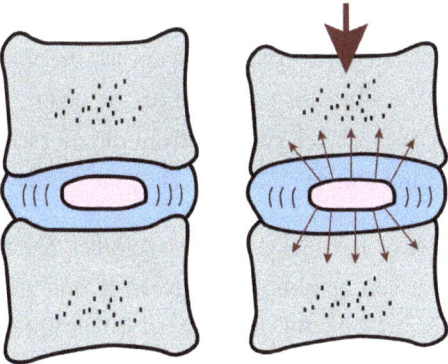

In the diagrams above, it is evident how the nucleus that is under tension reacts when loaded.

If we examine the mechanical properties of the disc, we will discover, in its simplicity, that it is nothing more than a shock absorber.

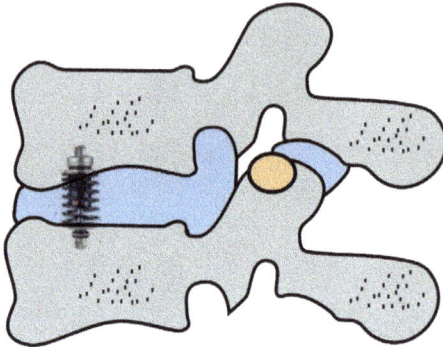

The Annulus is made up of layers and layers of rings that have a structure similar to that of an onion.

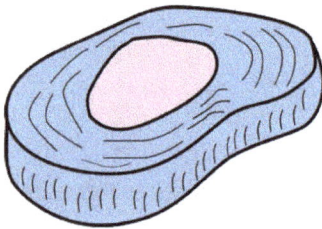

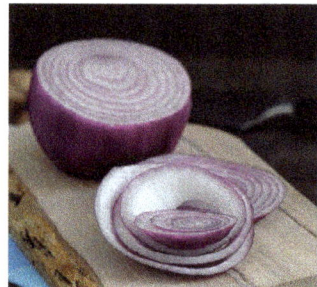

The only difference between the two, except for the shape and the smell, is the direction of the fibres in each one of the layers. In the onion, the fibres of each layer are parallel, running from the root to the stem, and this pattern is observed in all layers.

In the disc, the fibres of each layer are also parallel, like the onion, but the direction differs between neighbouring layers. If one layer has an oblique direction from right to left, the one next to it will have a direction from north to south (north being the head, south being the feet), and the third layer oblique from left to right, and so on. This way, the sum of all layers creates a strong net, and this strength is always maintained, even if the body is rotated.

This is because the different layers rotate accordingly. For example, the layer that was running from north to south in one rotation may run obliquely from right to left, and the neighbouring layer changes accordingly. This gives the same strength to the annulus in all potential positions the body takes and protects the nucleus in the same position and with the same properties.

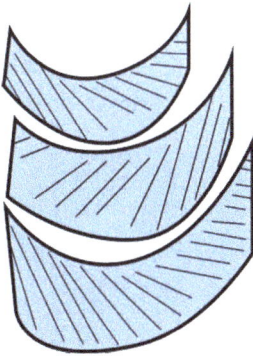

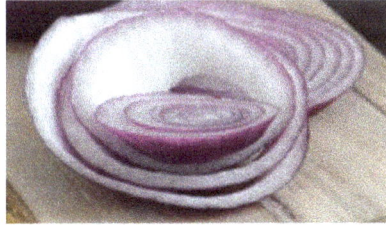

Unfortunately, as time goes by and with use, or to put it more accurately, misuse of the spine, the entire structure of the disc can become *"dehydrated."* In this case, the *"selfish"* nucleus *"sucks"* fluid from the neighbouring annulus in an attempt to maintain its shock absorption properties. As a result, the annulus becomes *"drier"* and more *"fragile."*

If an unusually excessive mechanical stress is applied to the back in this situation, the annulus may rupture and the disc under tension protrudes into the canal where the spinal cord and nerve roots are located. Depending on the extent of disc displacement and the severity of pressure on the nerves, neurological symptoms may arise. There are also instances where this disc dehydration occurs gradually, causing the space between the vertebrae to decrease under the weight of the body. These are referred to as *"degenerated discs."*

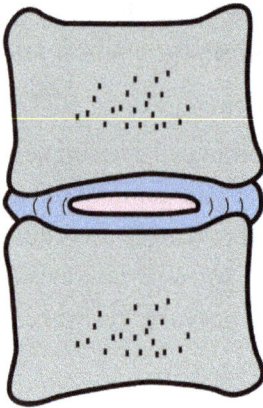

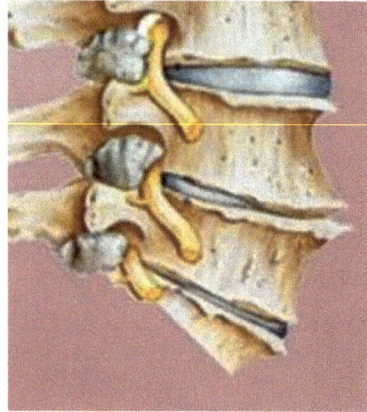

In the above diagram, the degenerative bulging disc is illustrated, where the nucleus becomes narrower and loses height, resulting in bulging discs. Imaging the disc as a deflated car tyre.

In the photo to the right, there is an artistic representation of narrow intervertebral spaces with the formation of osteophytes (extra bone *"spikes"*) at the superior and inferior parts of the vertebrae.

This latter picture indicates degeneration of the disc and the spine in general.

In cases where the disc is degenerative and bulging, meaning that it has lost height, there is an effect on the facet joint position, which is now *"subluxed"* (meaning that they are not in their ideal position), resulting in *"arthritic"* changes, as they are *"grinding"* their surfaces in these new positions. Think of these surfaces as two millstones that are slightly displaced and have to match their surfaces again. This procedure, however, creates some inflammation in the area.

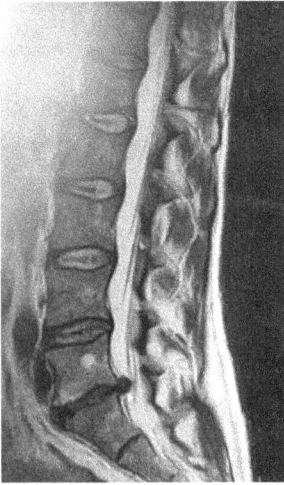

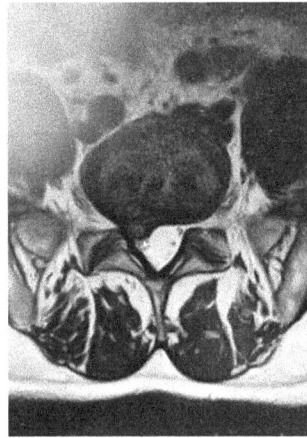

On the other hand, the scan on the right shows how the nucleus of the disc is penetrating to the left after breaking the annulus and pressing on the cord and possibly one of the roots.

Looking at the different pictures, you can understand why different movements could make your symptoms worse.

When you bend forward, in other words, moving into flexion, the posterior part of the spine and, at the same time, the intervertebral space opens and the front part of it is squashed. If there is a bulging disc protruding to the back, this protrusion becomes more prominent, so the disc compresses the nerves, increasing the pain and mainly causing pain in the legs.

On the other hand, when there is a great deal of wear and tear on the posterior joints and the extension of the intervertebral space, bending backwards makes the space narrower and the localised back pain becomes worse.

This is the reason why you need to know your pathology and how different positions need to be adapted according to the pathological findings during your intimate moments. Your condition has to be communicated with your partner.

Despite all this, it is known that not all the loads are absorbed by the bones and discs, but the muscles play a very significant role in offloading. They are not only there to move the bones but also to support them. These muscles can be considered as additional shock absorbers on their own. Think of them as sacks of fluid that are hermetically closed and have the ability to change the viscosity of this fluid. The higher the viscosity, the more resistance the structure has. In other words, the stronger the muscle is, the more load it can take on, which is something that everyone agrees with.

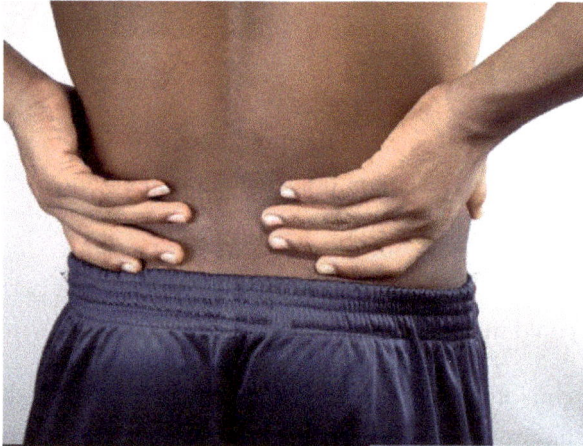

On top of that, the most important structure is a network of veins that exists all around the spinal cord and penetrates the bones. This network of veins is called the Plexus of Batson, as he was the one who described them. It is linked with the inferior veins that exist in the abdomen to the superior veins that exist in the thoracic cavity (chest).

These veins don't have valves like all other veins in our body. If we increase the intra-abdominal or intra-thoracic pressure, blood is driven to these veins and the flow can be from either direction.

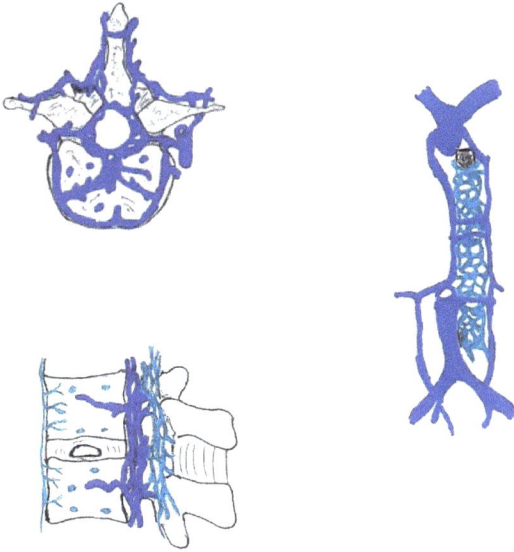

These diagrams show how the lower and upper main body veins are connected through a network called the Plexus of Batson, and how this network penetrates the bones.

The mechanical properties of this network can be easily explained by understanding the mechanism used for lifting heavy objects.

Imagine a weightlifting athlete in the Olympic Games and observe their movements and actions during preparation. You will notice that as soon as they are called, they powder their hands and tighten their belt very tightly. This increases the intra-abdominal pressure. Then, while preparing to lift, they take a deep breath and hold it. This increases the intra-thoracic pressure. By doing this, the diaphragm, which is a muscle that separates the chest from the abdomen, becomes immobilised under the pressure in both cavities. Similar actions occur at the pelvic floor. (Incidentally, weak pelvic floor muscles can lead to bladder leakage during weightlifting).

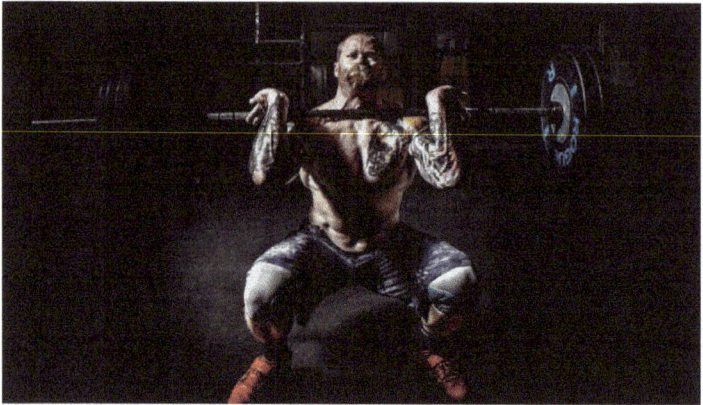

You can see in the picture below, that the veins around his neck are more prominent. This is due to increased intrathoracic pressure.

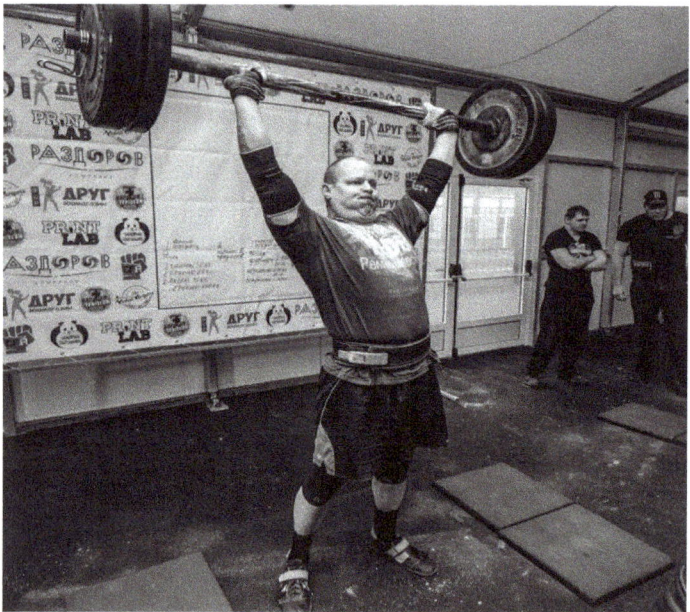

It is obvious how the athlete is holding his breath in the attempt to hold the weight over his head.

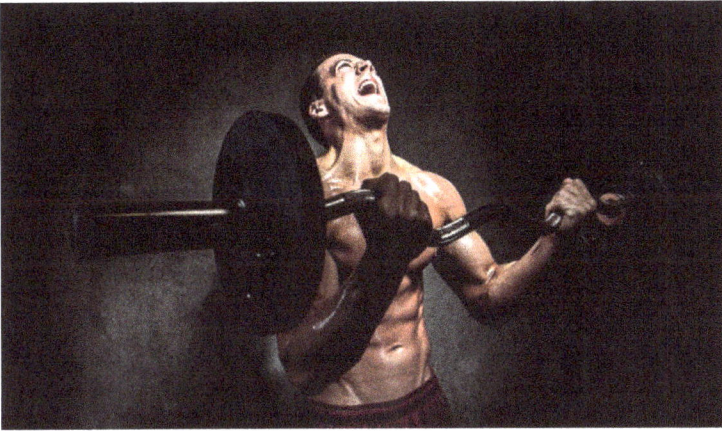

At the end of the successful lifting action, and while the weights are being lowered, a cry comes out of the mouth. This cry is a violent exhale of the held-in air.

You may ask, though, what is the reason for going through this description. It is simple. With all these actions, the athlete has pushed a vast amount of blood through this venous network, the Plexus of Batson, from both the abdomen and chest. The entire lifting process was done using a hydrostatic pressure mechanism assisted by a lever mechanism. It is the same way a heavy truck is lifted at the side of the road to change a flat tyre. Usually, a hydraulic jack is used in comparison to the means used to lift a sedan, where a jack made by arms and hinges applying mechanical lever mechanism principles is used because the car is lighter than the truck.

As it is obvious from these athletes, the human body can lift a great deal of weight. The majority of people are not aware of the exact number of loads that can go through our bodies every day during our daily activities. The forces applied to our muscles and joints are on a scale that sometimes the mind is not able to comprehend.

There are a number of scientists who have gone through and measured the loads that can go through different parts of the body, and this field of study is called Biomechanics.

When measuring the forces that go through our spine, you will be surprised. An experiment was conducted to calculate the loads going through our lower back. They used an individual of average weight and height and a weight of 20kg. This weight was positioned in different places and lifted in different ways. When the weight was placed in front of the individual's feet and they were asked to bend and lift it, they calculated that the load on the lower back was equivalent to 26kg. If the weight was lifted from the same position after the individual was asked to bend their knees and reach for it with a straighter back, the load was calculated to be 15kg. Then, they moved the weight to an arm's length position at a lower height and instructed the individual to lift it with an extended arm if possible. The calculated load was equivalent to 480kg.

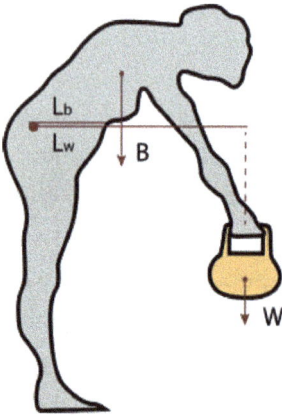

$$(L_b + B) + (L_w + W) = \text{Load (@ L5 - S1 spinal level)}$$

Thinking about the daily activities that anyone carries out, this latter position is used so many times during the day. For example, when a mother tries to save her child by lifting them from the ground while the child is running towards the stairs, or when a cook lifts a pot full of water from the back burner of the stove. In all these actions, a very high load is placed on the spine, and then everyone wonders why they end up with back pain.

Additionally, someone has to consider their own somatotype. The width of the body, when observed from the side, plays a role in the load put on the spine. The wider the body, the longer the imaginary moment arm on which the body weight is applied while someone is standing, resulting in greater force applied to the muscles around the spine, especially the posterior muscles.

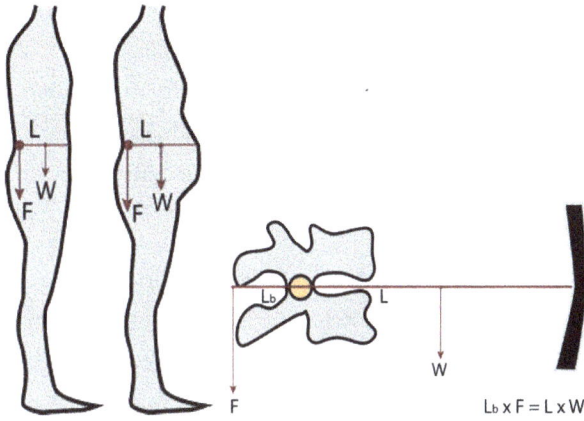

$$L_b \times F = L \times W$$

This is obvious in the diagrams seen above and how the forces can be calculated. The equation is simplified to the extreme, as other forces that can be applied to the body are not represented in the equation itself. It is clear that the wider the body, the higher the force used to keep us upright. In the case of a much wider body structure, the vector of the weight is moving forwards. If we use the example of a pregnant woman, the vector representing the weight can move considerably in front of the base of the body (in other words, in front of the feet), and there could be a tendency for the body to topple forwards. That is the reason why a pregnant woman's body changes standing position by hyperextending her spine (bending backwards), which can stabilise her as she stands.

Finally, as mentioned, discs are shock absorbers, but our muscles also have shock absorbing properties. So, stronger muscles can offload the spine and play a role in the viscosity differences mentioned above.

The shape and function of the spine can be influenced by other body pathologies. For example, hip problems such as arthritis and stiffness of the joint can make the symptoms of back pain more obvious because of a muscle that links the leg directly with the pelvis and the spine at the same time.

This muscle is called the Iliopsoas and is a combination of two muscles with different initial origins but a common attachment. These muscles are the Iliacus, whose belly is found on the inner side of the pelvis, and the Psoas, whose belly is attached to the small lateral processes and bodies of the lower vertebrae. Both bellies come together to form a united attachment with a common tendon on the inner side of the femur (thigh bone), close to the hip joint. One could simplify and say that this muscle is "linking the spine to the leg."

In the case of hip joint arthritis, the muscle could become stiffened and shortened in an attempt to protect and prevent extreme movements of the hip joint. This way, it pulls the spine forwards and has a crucial role in spinal loading. In the case of an individual suffering from back pain, there is a functional change in the spine and a potential increase in symptoms.

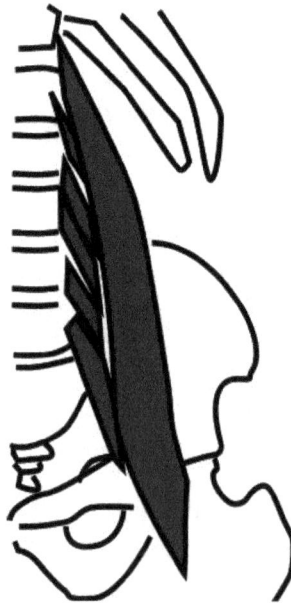

In summary, simple mechanical chronic back pain can be the result of one or many different causes that can affect a person. Understanding the mechanisms and function of our spine can help us comprehend our condition, and we could reflect by delving deeper to find out what initiated our individual issue and how we can approach it in the future.

Activity
Reflect and write down:

1. In your opinion, what is causing or making your back pain worse?

_____

_____

_____

_____

_____

_____

2. What remedies have you used to improve your symptoms?

_____

_____

_____

_____

_____

_____

HOW BACK PAIN AFFECTS PEOPLE

When back pain strikes due to physical trauma or tissue damage, as is the case with any trauma, it affects your entire body. There is an alarm that goes off in the brain, as it tries to comprehend what is happening. Emergency measures need to be put in place, and different channels of various functions are disrupted.

The only channel that remains active is self-preservation. The image you conjure is similar to that of a traumatised animal seeking isolation in its nest; humans also take the same action.

The first thing you do is find a safe corner and remain quiet. You do not want anyone to approach you. You do not want to move or speak; you simply want to be alone. In other words, you want to understand, analyse, and comprehend the situation, and then think and plan your next course of action.

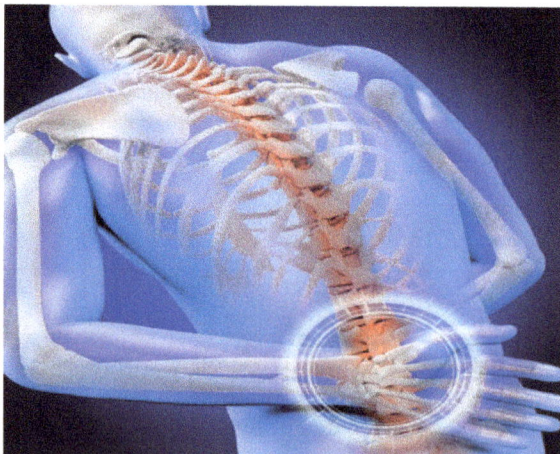

This is also the issue. Are you able to make the correct decision and act accordingly or not?

A number of questions need to be answered. These questions primarily stem from your own thoughts. They are thoughts that arise from past painful experiences that are resurfacing, and you are attempting to make sense of them. You analyse the situation from your own perspective. This can be confusing and potentially incorrect.

However, additional questions may arise from your surroundings, your loved ones, your extended family, and your friends. All of them are concerned about you, but their emotions impact you and contribute to the already "traumatised" mind.

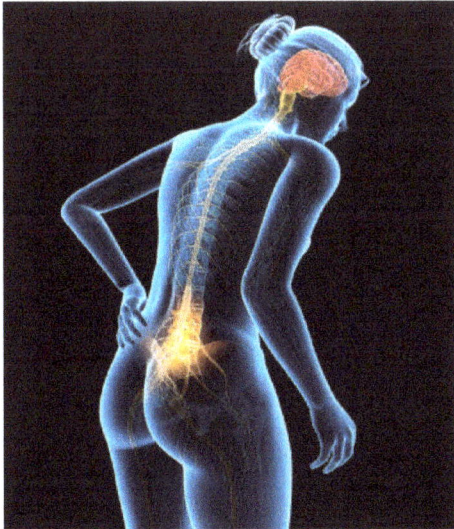

Your tendency to try to isolate yourself is affecting others in your environment even more, leading to different reactions and interactions between you and yourself, you and your immediate close family, or you and your extended family, as well as your friends.

Stress, anxiety, disruption of relationships, self-pity, and depression are some of the emotions that both you and the rest of your world are experiencing. You are trying to isolate yourself.

The only thing that you want from everyone, including yourself, is to be understood, informed, and supported.

We all know that back pain affects us in multiple ways. If we think logically, the original reason that initially influences us is damage to tissue. This could be a soft tissue (ligament, muscle, and disc) or the bone. I am excluding back pain that originates from other organs, such as the kidneys, pancreas, or vessels.

This initial damage creates an initial localised reaction which, with the help of the nerves, signals the central nervous system (spinal cord and brain) by providing information. As soon as this information is received, a generalised alert goes through the body, and the words "Brace-Brace," similar to when a plane is going to crash-land, fill our system.

This results in a loss of movement due to muscle spasm as the first mechanical reaction. The rigidity of the body, as the brain forces muscles to work in an attempt to eliminate movement, makes the muscles tired after a period of action. As muscles overwork, they require more blood supply to remove the waste they metabolically create with their constant activation. This extra blood supply creates more localised inflammation and swelling, resulting in more pressure, more pain, more painful signals sent to the brain, and more *"Brace-Brace"* demands.

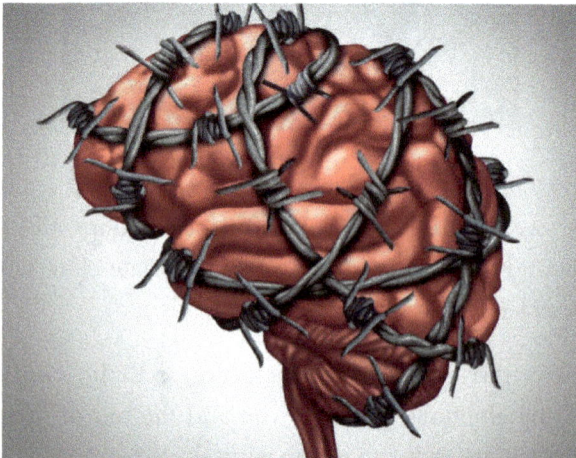

These demands are generated by the hypothalamus, which is part of the primitive brain. They affect the organs, particularly the adrenal glands that produce cortisol, a stress hormone. This leads to the production of "panic attack" hormones, which in turn affect the brain, other organs, and ultimately the pituitary gland. The pituitary gland, located at the base of the brain, is the master gland that communicates hormonal information to other glands and the cerebral cortex. This forms the initial cycle of panic.

If the pain persists for more than three months, it is classified as chronic. The brain remains in a state of alert due to hormonal influence, and a direct relationship between pain and constant stress response begins to develop.

Hormones play a crucial role in changing our behaviour, as panic-related information bombards the frontal cortex of our brain.

Studies have shown that daily activities are affected, which in turn impacts a person's morale. Uncertainty and anxiety gradually give way to depression, and the combination of immobility and depression affects the sufferer's social life. It is common to hear a sufferer say, "leave me alone." This altered social life leads to sleep disorders and problems in family relationships, among other things.

Moreover, as a person experiences these changes, it is discovered that depression, stress, and anxiety also affect hormone levels and can lead to additional symptoms such as sleep deprivation. When a lack of social life is added to all of these changes, the hormonal imbalance becomes more noticeable, creating an environment for further mental and behavioural disruptions.

The body and mind enter a state of problem acceptance and spiral downward, fuelling the pain and depression. This is the vicious cycle of chronic pain, where biology plays a small but constant role, mainly through its interaction with emotional factors.

The unfortunate consequence is that the disruptive behavioural changes of the sufferer directly affect their immediate family members, leading to changes in their own hormonal state. They too may find themselves in a state of panic. Their emotional state becomes strained, creating an emotional domino effect that eventually spreads to the wider community. This situation can result in numerous opinions and confusion.

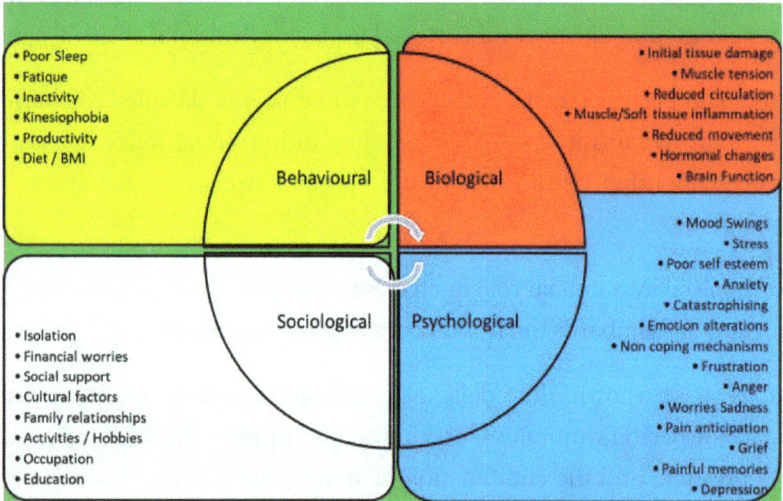

Behavioural
- Poor Sleep
- Fatique
- Inactivity
- Kinesiophobia
- Productivity
- Diet / BMI

Biological
- Initial tissue damage
- Muscle tension
- Reduced circulation
- Muscle/Soft tissue inflammation
- Reduced movement
- Hormonal changes
- Brain Function

Sociological
- Isolation
- Financial worries
- Social support
- Cultural factors
- Family relationships
- Activities / Hobbies
- Occupation
- Education

Psychological
- Mood Swings
- Stress
- Poor self esteem
- Anxiety
- Catastrophising
- Emotion alterations
- Non coping mechanisms
- Frustration
- Anger
- Worries Sadness
- Pain anticipation
- Grief
- Painful memories
- Depression

In the illustration above, it is clear how little space the physical *"problems"* occupy in comparison to the combined psychological, social, or behavioural *"problems"* that are affected by chronic back pain. The physical issues may be the initial presentation, but the rest are the result of various factors and stimuli accumulated over time.

To escape this complicated maze of physical and emotional troubles, you need to move in the right direction slowly and take each step carefully. Analysing the physical/biological aspect of the situation is necessary. The underlying tissue damage and its cascading effects lead to persistent pain behaviour.

It is already known that chronic low back pain affects more people on this planet than we can imagine, and as people age, the incidence increases. It is believed that 95% of low back pain symptoms have a *"mechanical"* cause, while only 5% are the result of generalised diseases.

Studies have found that people with low back pain, especially those with chronic symptoms, tend to avoid sexual activities out of fear that they may exacerbate their *"dormant"* symptoms. Additionally, they experience decreased arousal, reduced libido due to hormonal imbalance, and torment themselves with constant negative thoughts, leading to a loss of confidence. This is described as sexual disability, and about 60% of females and 85% of males experience such symptoms.

In addition to the physical and psychological issues these individuals face, certain medications, such as opioids or strong muscle relaxants, contribute to the negative clinical presentation due to their impact on the body's chemistry, and they further decrease sex drive.

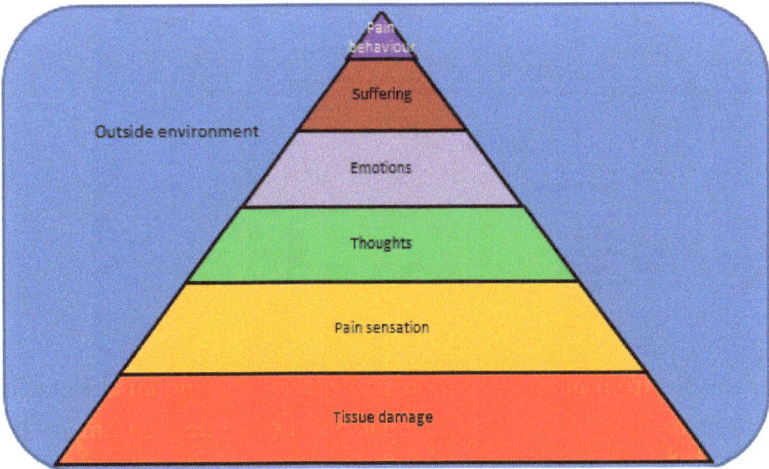

Even those who are attempting to engage in sexual activities report a 70% reduction in satisfaction, and approximately 60% decide to cease discussing these issues and cease communication with their partners. Although pain affects women more than men (90% to 70%), men are experiencing a higher prevalence of functional problems (82% of the population with back pain).

Influence of Back Pain Upon Intimacy

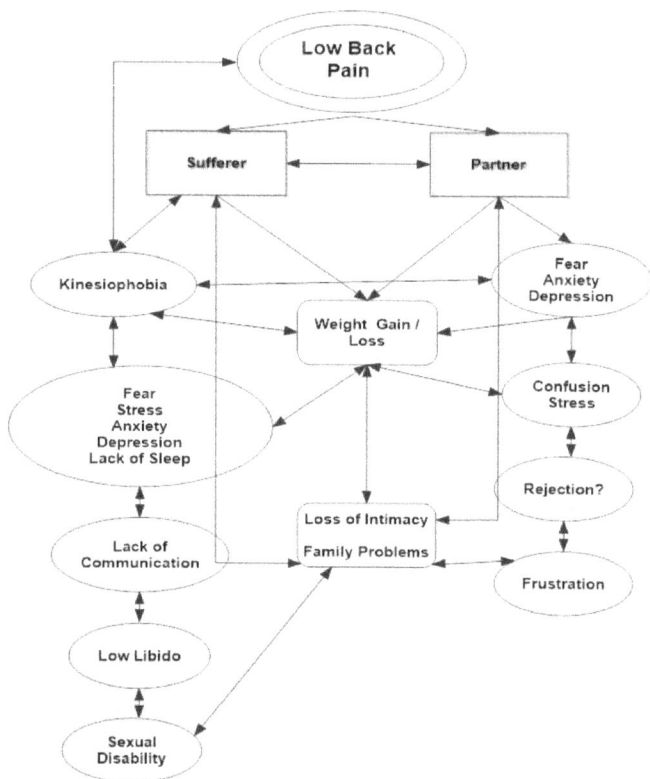

It is obvious from all the diagrams above that the emotional element is greater than any physical issues in a person who is suffering from low back pain. This has a direct effect on the surrounding environment and social circle, affecting the behaviour of a number of people. There are so many factors influencing each other and creating a very complex network that affects the lives of two people.

This is the vicious circle that you are going through when living a life with chronic low back pain: missing family activities, not being able to enjoy the laughter and company of your grandchildren, or not being able to do your hobbies and experience the close, tender touching of the most loved person in your life - your significant other. This is the reason we are here together, to walk the journey of reassurance, confidence management, and live a life of better quality.

From my professional experience, I can tell a story of a lady who presented with low back pain. The cause, following radiological investigations, was found to be two level bulging discs without any evidence of degeneration at the lower part of her spine. According to her history, the symptoms were getting worse after she had intercourse. Based on the description, she and her partner were using the *"missionary"* position, but her partner had the habit of grabbing and elevating her legs towards her chest, creating hyper-flexion of her pelvis and spine. It was at that time she experienced the most pain, but she was reluctant to do or say anything in case she could ruin his satisfaction. The symptoms remained present for about a week, slowly improving over time. Because of the pain and the fear, she was never able to feel pleasure herself. Having this experience, she avoided the activity, but at the same time, she was concerned about the future of her relationship. She came to me for stronger painkillers and further advice.

I sat down and explained to her the pathology and mechanisms of her spine, and how the same activity without hyper-flexion could give them both the same pleasure. I stressed that she must speak to her partner and explain the situation. In case she had difficulty communicating the problem, I offered to see them both and explain the issues.

It was obvious that communication, along with a lack of confidence, made her unable to stop that last manoeuvre. In my opinion, it was an act of dominance and not of satisfaction. I explained that he could feel the same satisfaction if he stopped doing it. Avoiding this last step would allow her to have the opportunity to feel pleasure herself, and become free of fear and guilt, as there would not be any anticipation of pain, as the pain would potentially be eliminated. The combination of the physical and emotional elements was affecting her ability to experience intimacy, and as a result, she felt concerned and guilty. She isolated herself because she was afraid to communicate and express her own feelings.

Due to the combination of issues she was facing and the severity of her depression, she made desperate statements about the future of their relationship.

The question is whether her mental state was affecting her symptoms. Literature states that depression and anxiety influence and amplify the symptoms of chronic low back pain. Her physical and mental state were working against her, and due to the constant hormonal influence on her central nervous system, her brain's chemistry was changing. Pain became her new reality, as she believed that it was the only way to live her life, even though it forced her to occasionally engage in activities she hated. Fear and pain dominated her, and the pain became deeply ingrained in her mind as the one thing that controlled her and altered her behaviour.

All of the above factors combined were impacting her social and intimate life, and the lack of these aspects increased her anxiety. She continued to cycle through this pattern, believing that the only way to break free was to increase her painkillers and avoid certain activities.

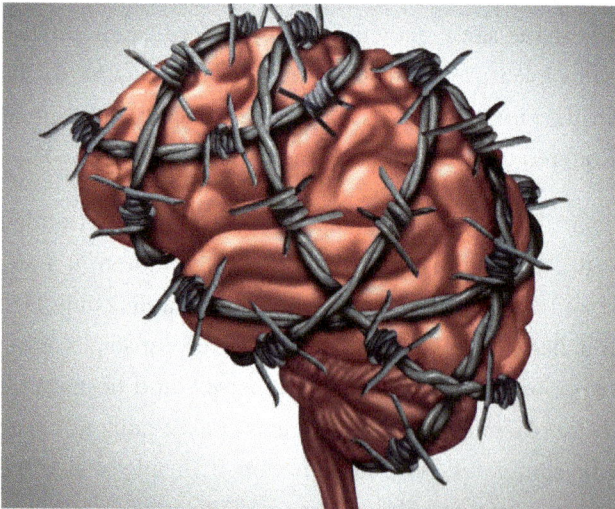

"CHEMICAL" EFFECT

Up to now, it has been demonstrated that patients' chronic pain influences their mechanical and psychological status. They fear that the pain, which is a part of their life, could destroy their future. They are focused on their pain, expecting to be *"hit"* by it again and again, which keeps them vigilant. Their anxiety levels are high, and they are constantly stressed. Only negative thoughts are pouring from their minds, and they develop kinesiophobia (fear of movement). They believe that if they move, the pain will come back, and the symptoms will worsen. This fear dominates their minds, and their entire being is immersed in a sea of uncertainty, anger, and desperation.

Because of this, they avoid everybody around them, and most importantly, they do not want to be touched in case that touch would make their pain worse. Fear dominates their mind.

This situation affects their stress hormones, which in turn affect the primitive part of their brain initially, the pituitary gland, and finally the frontal cortex of their brain where behaviour and emotions are stored. This is the end line on the emotional stage. The emotions are imprinted on their frontal cortex, creating new beliefs and habits. Once this is created, it is moved to the cognitive part of the cortex (the brain's archive). When this information is placed in the brain's archive, it influences the rest of the functional brain. People live as prisoners of their own brains, which dictate all the functions and thoughts of the body.

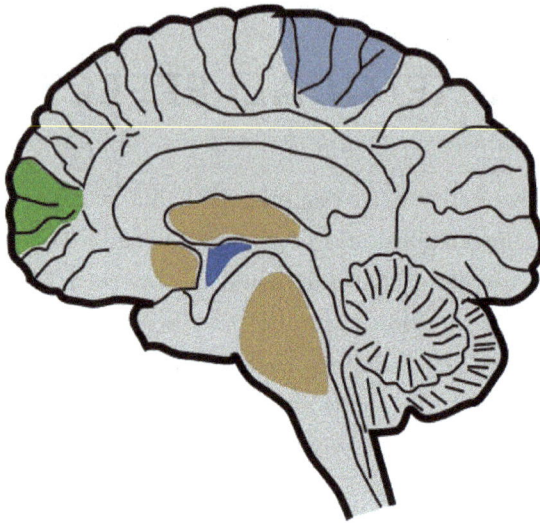

(The diagram above shows that the initial stimulus comes to the brown area (primitive brain – Brain stem, Hypothalamus, Amygdala) and via the purple (Pituitary gland) is influencing the green (Frontal cortex) and then mapped fully in the blue area (Cortical cognitive part) of the brain).

In other words, the majority of you who are suffering from chronic low back pain are starting to neglect yourselves. Cortisol, one of the stress hormones produced, is constantly bombarding the Hypothalamus and Pituitary Gland, the main central hormone controlling system, which are close to the primitive brain. From there, all the commands are flying in the body, resulting in complete derangement of the rest of the hormones. This way, Thyroxin, Dopamine, Insulin, and Testosterone are affected. The main way of influence is Cortisol, which reduces Dopamine. Dopamine then directly influences Thyroxin by reducing it. The reduced Thyroxin makes us more "relaxed," as it is trying to slow down our metabolism and fight back the effects of Cortisol. This imbalance also creates Insulin resistance and thus changes to your dietary behaviour, producing the environment for Type 2 diabetes as it drives you to consume more food. At the same time, it affects the *"inflammatory response"* of the body. With the activation of this cycle, we eat more as we try to affect our pleasure hormones, the endorphins, and thus it is called comfort eating.

All this activity results in weight gain. Extra weight, as we know, is a mechanical factor that increases the load on your spine. This extra load increases your symptoms of pain and adds more tissue reaction and inflammation. In addition, Insulin is responsible for further tissue inflammation, which can increase our symptoms. Because we are not getting better, our stress levels increase, more Cortisol is produced, and the cycle goes round and round. Testosterone, found in both males and females, is also influenced.

The reduction of Testosterone, due to increased Cortisol levels or opioid treatment, has an effect on libido, and so the sex drive is reduced. These changes in the body's chemistry create a lack of desire for any intimacy.

DOCTOR'S UNDERSTANDING AND LIMITATIONS

As doctors, we are trained to deal with science. We need hard data, proof, and measurements to carry on our lives. This is science to you. During our training, we are *"asked"* to super specialise, meaning that we are concentrating on a very narrow down field where we become experts, but we tend sometimes to forget the broader picture of the patient's needs.

This hyper-specialisation is great, and there is a need to give expert opinions in difficult cases for the benefit of the patient. But it is necessary to have a panel of doctors of different specialties to achieve this.

Sometimes, it is ignored that it is necessary to have a broader knowledge of medicine to allow us to see the person who came for help. A patient needs to be seen as a whole person and not only as a spine or as a leg or any part of the body you can choose. The patient is a human being and needs help in his or her entirety.

There are times that the Socratic quote *"I know one thing that I know nothing"* is definitely something that applies to us, as we may not know all the answers, and we must be mature enough to inform the patient about it. Say the phrase "I don't know" if necessary and ask for help.

But our "ignorance" may be part of our training. The tendency is to treat patients in a reactive conventional way and not a preventative or holistic one. We treat pain with painkillers, hypertension (high blood pressure) with hypotensives and so on, really giving numerous pills to our patients according to the symptoms we have in front of us. If there is even a minute indication, we offer surgery without thinking of any other way or solution to their problems.

In addition, there is this generalised perception that we as doctors must not talk about sex with our patients. This is a subject that has to be avoided due to cultural or political correctness. Ethically, this is correct if the illness the patient came to us has no relation to any pathology, physical or emotional, that would justify this kind of talk or questioning. This became a blanket covering all aspects, and in my humble opinion, we are denying treatment and solutions to our patients as we are not up to the level of their expectations.

During my training, I had the honour to work for about 18 months with a great Spinal Orthopaedic Surgeon. The weekly outpatient clinic had about 45 patients who were suffering from back pain at different stages, some in the beginning of their journey, and some already operated on or presenting problems months after their surgery. In our discussions, my mentor had said to me that it is expected to offer an operation only to 4% of the patients who are presenting themselves with back pain, even if they had neurological findings. The reason is that often these symptoms are improving on their own.

So, the offered treatments were mainly non-operative. If there was a need for an operation, it was offered only to people with neurological pressure that was not improving with any other means. It was made clear to them that the procedure is meant to relieve the pain that radiates to the leg and that they may experience permanent back pain due to the surgical scarring. I would "cruelly" explain all of this to the patients before their surgery as part of the informed consent. However, my training was solely focused on mechanical and physical solutions.

During my training years, I was never informed about the involvement of hormones in pain or how they influence the brain, our body functions, behaviour, and ultimately, our psychology. We were not allowed to discuss or question patients about anything related to *"sex."* It took the courage of a patient to bring up the topic during a consultation. Initially, I felt uncomfortable, as I was trained to feel discomfort whenever the word was mentioned. However, I overcame my initial reluctance and provided advice. I conducted my own research on the subject and discovered that sexual activity, which is a common part of human life, plays a significant role in patients' lives and the issues related to it. For this reason, I believe it would be necessary to inform them about these aspects in order to provide help in various aspects of their lives.

Activity

- Focus on the physical and mental reactions you had after seeing your physician and going through the treatment.

- How have your symptoms affected you?

_____

_____

_____

_____

- Concentrate on mental and emotional recovery by either exercising or engaging in mindfulness practice, in order to give your pre-frontal cortex a break from chaotic thoughts and emotions.

WAYS TO MANAGE YOUR BACK PAIN

What do you think a person who has been suffering from back pain needs in order to better manage the symptoms?

How can you resolve or improve the loss of intimacy?

Do you think that investigations, information, or surgery would be the answer?

On the other hand, is a better understanding of the cause and reason for the symptoms a better solution?

Do you think that a permanent solution to your back pain could be the answer?

Does a permanent cure or elimination of the back pain symptoms exist?

The real answer to these questions is complex. You will need more information, which can be obtained through a proper examination and, if necessary, further investigations. This would help determine the cause, and once the cause is known, a possible solution may become clearer. However, if someone is searching for a permanent solution to completely eliminate the symptoms, they are living in a utopian world. Once back pain has knocked on your door and become chronic, the word "elimination" should not exist in your vocabulary.

Now, by reading this cruel statement above, you may become more depressed and go hide in your dark corner. Your brain will be further alarmed as you were just told that the pain will be there at all times. Don't be disheartened, as the word "elimination" could be replaced by the word "management." I can assure you that the pain will not be there at every moment of your life. The best way to describe it is that pain has the ability to visit you sometimes, but you will be given the armamentarium to fight it back and stay on top of it. Think that you have the ability to turn the volume down, and it is up to you to learn how much pain you will allow your body to have.

You need to stay active on many levels, and all is achievable.

Firstly, the body's muscle movement. Being mobile represents a healthy being that is not afraid to move. A body that can be used for daily activities and thrive. A body that is given to us by our Creator and something we need to cherish. There is an ancient Greek quote by Aristotle: *"Healthy mind in a healthy body."* This tells us that if you look after your body, you are also looking after your mind, as these two interact. To create a healthy body, we need to:

- Keep moving and exercising.

- Take care of the fuel you put into your body. Nutrition is key. Nutrients include not only the physical food you digest, but also the thoughts you feed your brain too.

- Plan ahead and stay committed. If you find it difficult to stick to your plan, enlist the help of someone else such as a trainer or a family member, to keep an eye on your progress.

- Do not fear movement.

- Do not be afraid of engaging in intimate activities, as it has been found that they can help you get in shape.

The more you get in shape, the more confident you become, and your brain becomes more active and content. Confidence gives you a sense of self-assurance, reduces feelings of fear and self-doubt, and eliminates worrying thoughts. When you are confident, you also feel more motivated. Exercise can help your brain release endorphins, hormones responsible for your happiness.

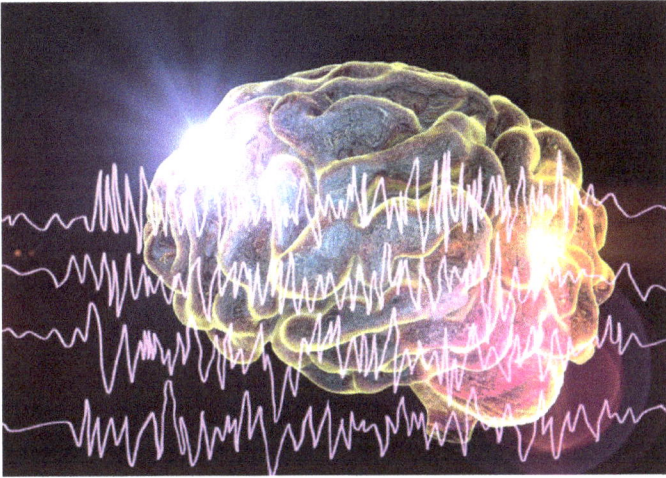

Following this, it is necessary to focus on solving the problems by removing any negative thoughts and striving to reach your goal with a positive attitude. To achieve this, you need to become mentally aware of your issues, concentrate, and find ways to help you achieve your purpose, which is managing your back pain and finding ways to experience forgotten pleasure.

Protecting your mind, wellbeing, and enjoying intimacy are the subjects of your purpose, so you need to be dedicated to nurturing your powerful and beautiful thoughts. Keep moving forward at all times, plan for the future, and have confidence that you will resolve the issues.

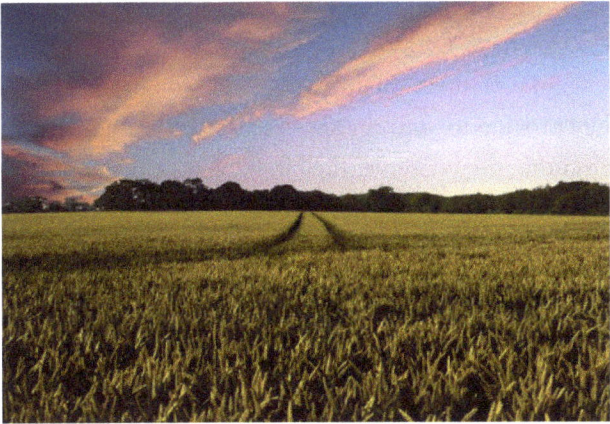

Do not feed your mind with fear, doubts, worries, stress, and anxiety by saying that you cannot succeed in controlling your symptoms. By being happy, optimistic, and certain of your successful outcome, you are also influencing your partner's emotions. Happiness and confidence are contagious.

Repair the relationships. Be close to your significant other, discuss any worries, communicate, and work together to find solutions. Connect with your loved one. Develop better and stronger relationships with this important person who is ready to help you if they were aware of the issues. You have to keep your loved ones close and allow them to assist you on your journey. This is the only way for you to be supported and understood.

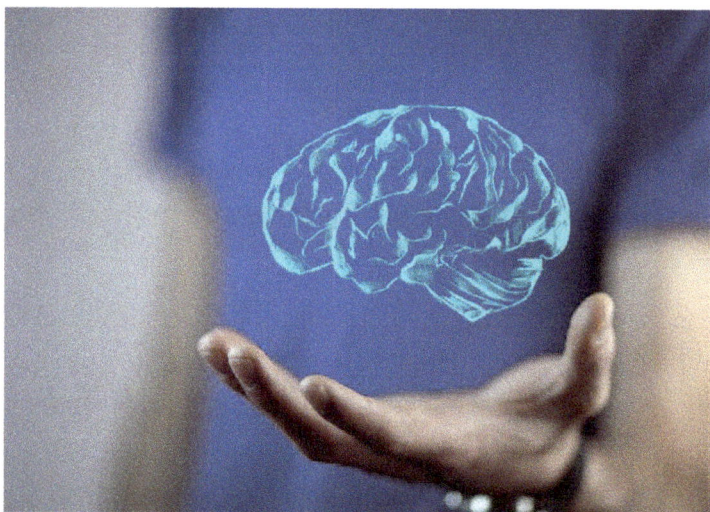

Fall in love again with them. Being with people you love and appreciate for the help they provide to you can also release endorphins. By giving them back the gratitude they deserve, the circle of happiness is whole. On the other hand, you become so powerful, passionate, and protective of your wellbeing that persons who are creating any feelings of anger, sadness, anxiety, depression, and other negative thoughts are removed from your horizon. It is known that you do not have any great control over others, but you can control yourselves. Therefore, by the power of your mind, you eliminate the toxic negative environment around you.

You need to be aware of your actions, so you need to plan ahead. You need to prearrange everything that can affect the time you have to spend with your partner. This way, you remove the chances of anxiety and any negative worrying thoughts, as you have already planned all the positive things you need to do.

You need to find ways to balance the actions of your life. The majority of people forget about family, and in doing so, they lose contact. Try not to do that, as it will create confusion for you. It is good to focus on balance. Your environment has to be balanced. You have to be balanced. You need to become confident again. Lack of confidence can create anxiety and stress. You must communicate with your significant other and work together; trust one another. By using communication, you can achieve a solution to any issues. If there is still a problem, try together to find the final answer. Become positive, confident, and create an overall greater future.

In summary, movement is the beginning of the physical actions that can provide you with motivation and confidence. However, understanding and communicating your issues and carefully planning the correct path together with your partner will guide you to the goal of finding together the way to achieve sensual and sexual pleasure without any fears and questions about tomorrow. Commit yourself to the purpose of making your intimate moments once more joyful, full of love, respect, and relaxation, instead of anxiety, fear, and worries about the return of the pain.

Embrace the Epicurean quote *"What is good is easy to get, and what is terrible is easy to endure,"* meaning that a smile or a nice word (the good) is easy to receive or give, and every challenge is an opportunity to win; don't complain.

MOTION

The first thing the brain does when the body is in pain and in a state of emergency is to order immobilisation. The condition of kinesiophobia (fear of motion) develops. This order, given from the brain to the rest of the body, is led by fear. You need to fight this. It is known that movement or better yet, exercises, can make you happy as the brain releases endorphins. The easiest way to treat this is to start with short walks. The initial walk could be around the yard, around the block, or a stroll down to do some window shopping. The frequency can gradually increase and become a daily routine.

As energy levels increase, the distance can increase and slowly some exercises may be added. These exercises can include initial stretching and rotational movements of the torso but can gradually increase in complexity and frequency.

Increased movement gives you the confidence that motion is not bad, and this way you can treat your kinesiophobia. If there is an opportunity to join a gym or do exercises in water, like aqua aerobics or swimming, it would be very beneficial. Don't forget that when you are in water, gravitational loads on the joints are lesser. So water is very beneficial.

The exercises have to take into consideration the function of the different groups of muscles and the direction of their fibres.

Many consider sexual activities as a great form of exercise, as this motion is linked with emotions. They call it sexual therapy. It is found that muscles get stronger, and the body improves posture. This result is due to the boost of sexual confidence and the belief that all is possible, as your emotions that bring you happiness are high due to the elevated levels of happy hormones within your bloodstream. Endorphins are not the only hormones you are producing, but oxytocin, serotonin, and dopamine are elevated too, resulting in the suppression of cortisol and insulin that create inflammation and pain. Testosterone is also increased. It is found that the latter controls pain and helps the brain feel it less, while also improving your sex drive.

In other words, motion is the key factor in our attempt to stimulate our brain and make it not fear movement. Sexual activities help in these grounds.

MUSIC - MOVIES

Art is evident in its clear influence on our emotions. The most well-studied art is music, and secondary to that are movies, as they combine visual and acoustic stimuli. Music combines rhythm, harmony, pitch, melody, and meter.

Music is one of the means that, since our young age, makes us happy, relaxed, and mobile. Our mothers know this well. It is a form of stimuli that influences our brain, mainly in the emotional sphere.

You have favourite tracks that make you move and dance quietly even when you are on your own as soon as you hear them. There are other tracks that make you stay silent and delve deep in an attempt to find the roots of your thoughts, and those that may help you go to sleep.

Don't forget that in the beginning of our lives, our mothers were singing lullabies to help us fall asleep.

Music influences your brain in more than one area. It affects not only the ancient brain but also the secondary brain. The specific areas involved include the insula (yellow), hypothalamus (red), amygdala (dark blue), and prefrontal cortex (brown).

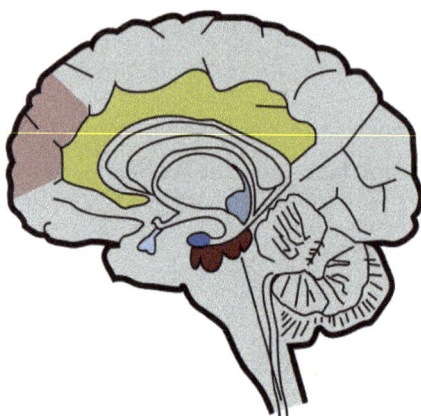

The hypothalamus and amygdala are part of the ancient brain. The hypothalamus controls body temperature, hunger, thirst, and mood, and it directly influences the pituitary gland (light blue) and, through it, all the other glands.

Through the secretion of multiple hormones, your metabolism can be changed, as well as the frequency of your pulse, appetite, awareness, and behaviour. All these hormonal changes and their effects on your functions are directly linked to the circles, loops, and logical sequence of the waves that the rhythm, tone, acceleration, and intensity of music create.

The main hormones that are produced are oxytocin, arginine-vasopressin, and endorphins, which are primarily produced in the hypothalamus and pituitary gland, and dopamine, which is produced in the adrenals. Dopamine is responsible for a person's good mood. All these hormones directly influence our emotions as well as other hormones and can alter our metabolic status.

Oxytocin, as well as dopamine, suppress cortisol (also produced by the adrenals), which can reduce anger, stress, anxiety, and depression. Arginine-vasopressin influences and reduces cardiac rhythm and blood pressure. Dopamine can also affect thyroxin (hormone that plays a role in activity/alertness) and insulin (hormone that controls blood sugar) by reducing them, while testosterone (androgenic hormone that also plays a role in activity/alertness) is increased. It has been found that testosterone can control pain.

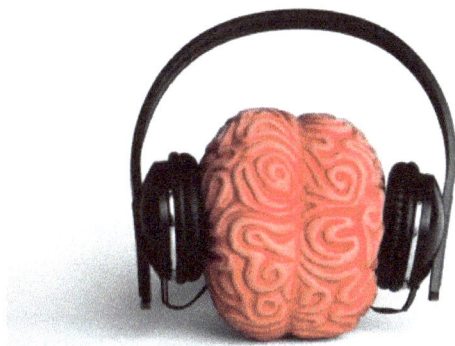

Soft, easy-listening music or gentle classical music has been found to increase oxytocin, endorphins, arginine-vasopressin, dopamine, and testosterone, while decreasing thyroxin and insulin. This way, we can calm down and improve our mood, becoming more positive for the future.

On the other hand, hard rock, and punk music, as well as classical music from certain composers like Wagner, for example, have the opposite effect on us, putting us in a state of alertness. This is the reason that soft music would not be very helpful in case of driving long distances, although it can be very good if we are in a traffic jam, as it helps us lower our stress levels.

Researchers claim that easy listening music alleviates the psychological states of anxiety, tension, and stress in individuals.

Based on all of the above, we can consider music as an alternative "medication" to decrease the factors that amplify the symptoms of sufferers from chronic low back pain.

During intimate moments or foreplay, music is found to be a key factor that can improve moods and assist in arousal, as it has a direct effect on hormonal secretion. All happy hormones are found to be elevated, but the final state of excitement during the act is driven by testosterone, as this hormone is found in both males and females.

Similar effects are observed with the type of movies we watch. Researchers conducted an experiment by dividing a group of individuals into three sub-groups. The first group had to watch romantic family films or comedies, the second group watched action and horror films, and the third group watched documentaries. The hormones of all individuals were measured before and after the films. They found that the first group had low stress hormones due to high levels of dopamine and testosterone, resulting in people feeling calmer, similar to the effect of listening to easy listening music. The second group had raised stress hormones, while the third group showed no difference between their two readings.

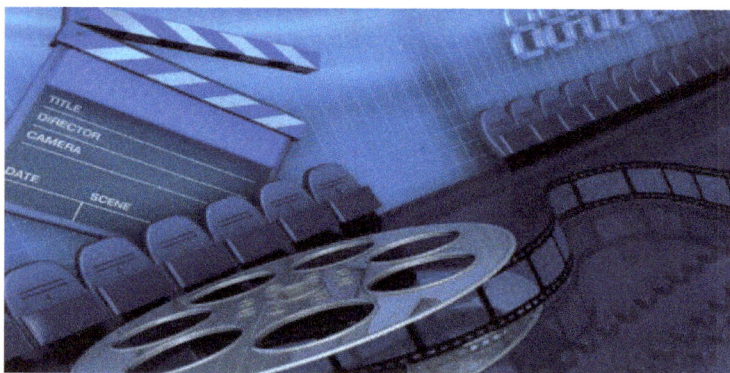

In summary, it is better for you to listen to easy listening music and soft classical or watch romantic films and comedies, as they help reduce our stress levels and anxiety. It is necessary to avoid Punk Rock and Horror films if you want to become calmer.

So, music is a practice that can be used for your benefit to alleviate your *"misery."*

MEDITATION

Another way to control and train the mind and moods is through meditation. This can involve a combination of music and movement or even the absence of both. The purpose is to help the mind focus and concentrate on positive thoughts and goals that everyone has. I can tell you that by visiting favourite places, you may be aided in becoming calmer. By being calm, you can follow practices that help you stay focused on a specific task and train the mind to have a positive outcome. During meditation, high levels of Serotonin are measured.

You can practice meditation in a quiet room or by listening to music indoors or outdoors. Some people prefer to be in specific spots in nature or concentrate by doing specific exercises, like yoga.

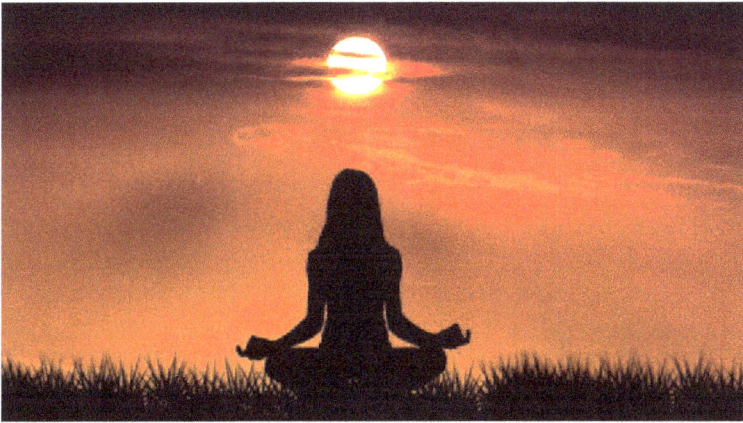

To have the desired positive effect, someone needs to develop a strong belief in an idea or desired outcome and react positively in an attempt to remove any existing obstacles. Concentration on the present goal and visualisation, while controlling your physical reactions, is necessary. Strong focus on the purpose in the present moment, without judgement or fear about anything you may encounter in your future life. Deep concentration within the mind itself is necessary and can be achieved by using all mental and physical power to focus on that specific belief and feel in your mind that it is happening.

As mentioned, in most cases, the use of soft music or a tranquil environment can help with concentration.

Part of the sensual preparation and foreplay, especially during massaging from your partner, involves a *"deep retrieval"* from the surrounding environment, where you concentrate only on the present moment. This can also be considered an act of meditation.

MENTAL AWARENESS

Mental awareness is a constant work in progress for refining our goals; it is not a one-time process. It is something you need to repeat frequently as your circumstances change. You need to use it to clarify things for yourself and plan your actions. This way, you will avoid any distractions from your environment or even from your own self.

There are some steps you need to take:

1. Reflection: You need to be able to analyse the state you are currently in, pinpoint it and find out what is influencing it.

2. Love yourself: Be kind and calm with your emotions and feelings. Imagine the life you want and dream of having and embrace it. Plan for it and live for this future "ideal but realistic" life. Fill your mind with happy emotions. If you are in a dark place, you are becoming numb and staying there only because you are "living in the moment" and imprisoning yourself within it, becoming unable to come out of it. Do not dwell on painful memories or fear any change. The majority of our fears are not real or useful. Become a positive person.

3. Control: Become disciplined and persist in the goals you set for yourself to achieve. Be able to control yourself. *"A man who cannot control self is not free."* - Pythagoras. So become free.

4. Flow: Become able to create a path that is so well defined that actions and thoughts will flow freely, like water flowing from the river to the sea.

5. Willingness to improve yourself: To achieve it you need to think intensely about the ideal future destination and believe in this

new change you are planning for your life. Love this change, become enthusiastic about it, dream of it and be happy about it. Do not look back to the dark life. Create a strong will to improve your life one step at a time and continue progressing.

After considering all of the above, it is crucial to plan, work hard, and stay on the right track. You should begin by assessing your current condition and accepting it.

It is important to acknowledge the existence of back pain as a fact. It may take time to fully understand and accept that back pain is a long-term condition, and the only option is to confront it and enhance your quality of life without fear.

Depression and anxiety caused by physical issues are recognised and acknowledged.

The future objective should be envisioned. The path you need to follow in order to achieve your goal should be carefully considered and designed.

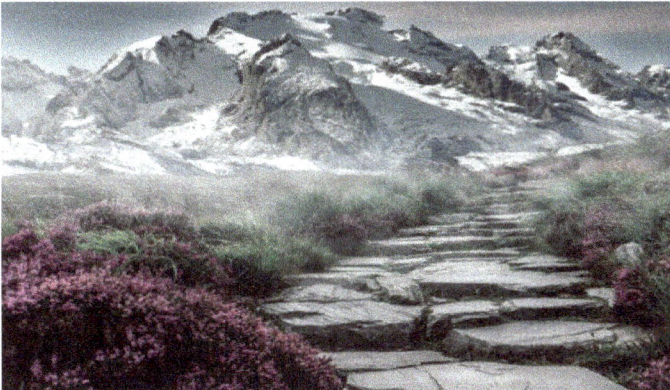

The path is nicely paved with slabs, and you have to walk on them, stepping on them one step at a time. Follow this path, focusing on your purpose. The direction has to be clear and focused on the goal. Reverse engineering can also be used to help you achieve your arrival at your destination. Imagine that you have already been to your desired spot. Then, turn back and see the path you have walked, and you can track all the steps you need to take on your way to our future goal.

You know that you need to follow this road step by step and one step at a time, and only in this way will you reach your ideal outcome. The need to analyse the reasons you have that drive you to this change is paramount. You need to know why you need to change. Then you need to answer what you have to do to achieve the change and, therefore, achieve your goal.

The thought that is planted in your mind has to be so intense that it will create a new behaviour pattern, like the groove water can create on the rock. The deeper the groove, the more efficient it is, and it is easy to be filled with more water, facilitating the flow of it to the river and, ultimately, the final destination. The more frequent and more intense the thought is, the deeper the "groove."

Your goal is to strengthen all your new thoughts with repetition and perseverance, and in this way, you are supporting your behavioural change.

You must not be afraid if there are times when you find yourself in a situation that is not preferred. You are not a loser. Create this mental picture. When you want to learn how to dance, you go to a dancing instructor and ask them to teach you the moves. When you learn them, you are asked to go to the fair and dance in front of all the people. It will be normal to step on some toes or even lose the steps or the rhythm, but you persevere and insist to dance. This way, you start becoming an expert.

There are people who say that they don't need an expert to show them the ways to improvement. Is this a sound attitude? If you want to play the guitar, and you don't go to an instructor, then the only thing you learn to do is noise. You must remember that if you don't want to be instructed by an expert in the field, you may have a potential issue with criticism.

Aristotle preached that to have well-developed mental awareness, you need to firstly recognise your own feelings and be able to manage them, and secondly, be able to recognise the feelings of your fellow humans and be able to be flexible so as not to offend them.

By saying this, you have to become able to understand yourself, find your goal, your destiny, and make sure that you know why you want to be there. Plan your way, start your journey by figuring out how you will do it. If you are not clear about how to do it, find someone who has made the journey, and he/she will help you manage it with their help if necessary. They may also help you be accountable for your actions. This is my role. I am here to assist you and share my experiences; this way you will thrive to a better quality of life by managing your back pain better.

Planning, repetition, and perseverance are helping you to develop confidence and motivation for your future achievements. All of these also influence, on the other hand, your hormonal balance.

Hormones and emotions interact as explained, meaning that the frontal cortex has new imprints and thus creates new habits. In other words, you need to get in a state of happiness. I am not implying the use of "chemistry" for that, as I am against any medicinal help.

It is found that achieving happiness is not a passive path, but you need to act upon it. Real happiness is not linked to material possessions. It is mainly something that you live and experience. Certain activities can easily drive you to happiness. Typically, you need to concentrate on something that is very interesting to you and occupies your brain fully. You need to have fun during these activities. You need to enjoy what you do, and this way, you help your spiritual wellbeing.

Pleasurable activities, such as social gatherings and creative pursuits, such as achievement of goals, increase your confidence. Confidence increases your enthusiasm, and you become more motivated. Being enthused and motivated creates happy emotions, and this way, you stimulate your frontal cortex. This influences your overall behaviour, and you become more positive. Your change can influence the pituitary gland, and thus, your whole hormonal system. It is well known that after physical activities, a person is more content, relaxed, has a positive attitude, and becomes confident, so they can overcome all obstacles due to the overflow of endorphins within the body circulation.

You need to find ways to engage your mind and body and ensure that you have a clear dream that you want to materialise, and remember that the treasure exists within you. Don't search elsewhere. Follow Dr. Daniel Amen's (renowned neuropsychologist with international acknowledgments) words; you have to destroy the ANTs (Autonomous Negative Thoughts) that poison your brain and eat away at your treasure. Love your brain and protect it.

Reviewing the aforementioned subjects as the starting point, the destination, the reasoning, and the how you will achieve the goal and change, ensure that they are questioned and answered within you, and your brain and thoughts have to be protected.

Analyse your habits and focus on the necessary actions for a positive outcome and the elimination of any negative thoughts. Eliminate any distractions.

Concentrating on this transformation, believe in yourself and act as if there is no problem. After acknowledging that the back pain is there, but your confidence is elevated to such levels that it influences your mind in a highly positive way, driving you towards your new goals. The belief and feeling that you will experience the most amazing intimate moment with your significant other. Once this behaviour fills your inner self, you will notice a change in your partner's behaviour. Your transformation is transmitted to the other person, who becomes more positive and gets closer to you. Understanding your limitations, emotions, and needs is essential, as is communicating them effectively. You will find that respect, protection, love, and action according to your wishes will come pouring towards you. Your transformation is improving your relationship as positivity fills the space you are floating into.

Please do not forget that this is only for educational purposes. If you have any health issues, please consult your own doctor for further advice and treatment. This is not a medical consultation.

Activity

From all the previous activities you have undertaken, you must already know a lot about your current state, the treatment methods you have followed, and your goals. Now, you need to bring all of this together and delve deep into yourself to answer the following questions:

1. Where are you now and what is stopping you?

_____

_____

2. Where do you want to go and what dreams do you have?

_____

_____

3. Why do you need to do this?

_____

_____

4. What do you have to do to achieve this change?

_____

_____

5. How will you do it?

_____

Once you are calm and settled, choose one goal to pursue and stick with it.

WAYS OF TRANSFORMATION

Allow me to use my experience as a bridge that brings to you the solution, the resurrection as I call it and describe how I found ways to manage all the difficulties my patients faced.

Anyone who has an *"unknown"* problem initially panics and sinks into the dark abyss. I know that a lot of you are going through these dark experiences, so please allow me to offer myself and my services, so I can help you overcome this negativity, come out of the abyss, and become able to return to the light.

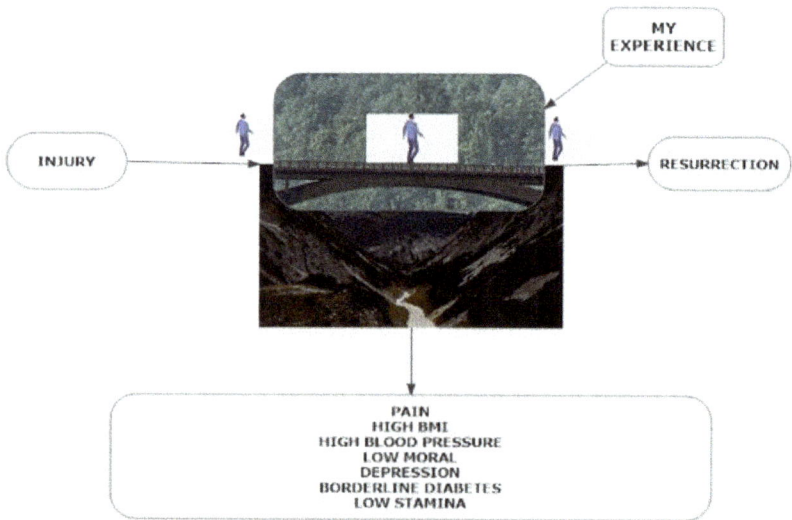

I am here to share my experiences and serve you based on the following factors. Firstly, I can help you through my professional experience as an Orthopaedic Surgeon for the past 39 years. Through extensive research and experimentation, I have managed to improve the symptoms of those seeking help, specifically addressing issues they face during their intimate moments.

When suffering from chronic low back pain, the ultimate goal is to control it and live a normal life, ideally without symptoms. However, it is unfortunately not possible to completely eliminate symptoms. Therefore, the realistic goal is for you to live a life with long periods of normality, free from symptoms, and be able to experience pleasure without fear.

I am here to share my experiences, strategies, the steps my patients have taken under my guidance, and the proposed solutions that anyone can implement to improve their overall health - physically, mentally, and sexually.

Once more, I am stressing that all the information given is based on my own experiences and serves an educational purpose. You should only keep the sections that resonate with you. Please note that this is not a medical consultation or advice.

MOTION

Generally, when you are suffering from low back pain, you need to stay mobile. You need to fight the potential increase in your weight, and as mentioned, movement helps increase your body's flexibility and the secretion of happy hormones. You must not make any excuses like, "I never have time." This latter statement is the silliest excuse someone can have. I urge you to forget this phrase. YOU HAVE AND YOU MUST MAKE TIME FOR YOURSELF. Your doctor may be necessary to give you medications to improve your pain, but you are the captain of your ship. You have to take responsibility and be certain that you will help yourself.

Initially, walking may be the simplest movement you need to do. Buy a pair of trainers with shock-absorbing soles and insoles. Don't forget that discs are shock absorbers, and they need assistance. This external shock absorption also helps other joints. Initially, your walks will be short, and gradually the distance will increase.

When you find that you are getting comfortable with this level of motion, and because your enthusiasm may start to fade, try to find ways to persevere and sustain the activity. You may need to subscribe to a local gym. Initially, gentle exercising and swimming could be your goal, but gradually the level of activity will increase, so step by step, you will improve your motion. Walking in water may be a good starting point, as gravity is reduced. Many people attend aqua aerobic classes. This helps boost your self-confidence and self-esteem.

In the following pages, you will find possible beneficial exercises that can be followed by someone who is suffering from low back pain. These exercises help anyone achieve their goal of improving muscle strength and supporting the back.

Why do you need to stay mobile? Movement helps with your thinking, confidence, and the hormonal system of your body.

What is the goal? Mechanically, you need to become more flexible and be able to use the muscles as additional shock absorbers and stabilisers of your spine. To stabilise your spine, you need to have strong core muscles. Flexibility, on the other hand, needs to be extended not only to the spine but also to the hip joints, as the upper part of the thigh bone (femur) is attached to the spine by muscles, with the most important one being the iliopsoas, as seen in the drawing.

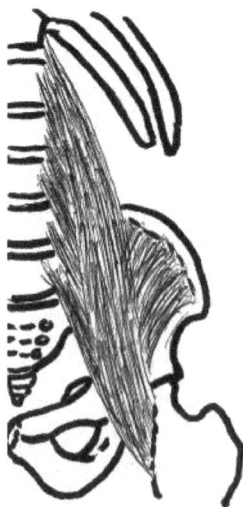

When people hear about core muscle strengthening exercises, they often focus solely on the abdominal muscles, specifically the 6-pack muscles known as the rectus abdominis. However, it is important not to overlook the lateral abdominal muscles, which have fibres that run in oblique or horizontal directions. Crunches, which target the front abdominals and their top-to-bottom fibre orientation, are insufficient on their own. To achieve overall strength, a combination of exercises that involve all the muscles is necessary.

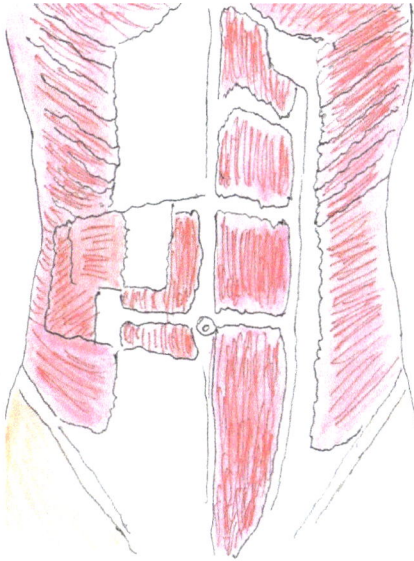

So, what kind of exercises do you need to do? How often do you need to do them? Which muscles are involved in each exercise? What are the overall benefits? What time of day do you need to do them?

There is a specific way to prepare for your exercises. First, you need to learn to concentrate on your breathing. Then, you need to warm up and follow a sequence of stretching and working out.

Why is breathing important, you may ask?

For the following reasons:

1. You need oxygen to reach your muscles during your workout.

2. Your mind and body work together, so relaxation is fully understood by your brain, and this helps with the release of muscle tension when necessary. (Breath in = tension of muscles, breath out = relaxation).

3. When the body has less air in the lungs, it becomes more flexible, although the muscles are not well oxygenated.

4. You are getting into a rhythm, as breathing can become "music in your ears."

To perform any exercises and increase the muscle response, you need to warm up. A warmed muscle is more flexible. You are fighting stiffness, so you need flexible muscles. This technique helps the blood flow through the muscles. Warming up could be done with simple light exercises or simple movements. In some cases, a warm bath could be considered.

Stretching gives flexibility to the muscles, so it is essential before you do any strengthening exercises. A stretched, flexible muscle can move a greater distance than a short, stiff muscle. Additionally, a short, stiff muscle is prone to injuries as the range of motion is limited. An injury caused by overstretching a stiff, short muscle can result in prolonged symptoms, such as worsening back pain in some cases. When you exercise and stretch your muscles, it would be beneficial to maintain the stretched position for five to ten breaths.

Now, let's talk about frequency. Initially, it is evident that you have to start light, and you could divide some of the exercises in the morning and some before bed. This way, you may find that you will achieve good results. In both cases, a warm bath or shower will help with muscle recovery and provide a better night's sleep after the evening session. Please do not overdo it.

When your mobility improves and you start the strengthening exercises, it is better to perform them once every three days. This will give your muscles enough time to recover.

So now let's focus on some of the exercises. Wear comfortable clothing.

Below, you will find some exercises you can do at home (you will need a well-padded yoga mat).

Exercise is known as another type of potential exercise, and this is the reason for writing this book. It not only helps your muscles but also improves hormone secretion and mental health.

In the following pages, you can see some of the most common exercises for improving back pain, but please imagine how you can incorporate some of them during sexual activities. Don't forget that warming up, in this case, means taking a warm bath prior to intimate activity or massaging with oils. In some cases, you can use medicinal creams.

Terminology

Isometric: a muscle contraction without resulting in movement.

Isotonic: a muscle contraction producing movement.

Dorsal area: the back of the body.

EXERCISES

The following exercises are generally simple. You can perform them in your own home, using your own furniture and even wearing your everyday clothes. You don't have to own any specific equipment or be a member of any expensive club.

In case you want to wear comfortable clothes or have a yoga mat or even go to the gym, I will not fault you. It will be much more comfortable, and I understand. Please do what is best for you.

The photos illustrate the sequence of positions you have to take.

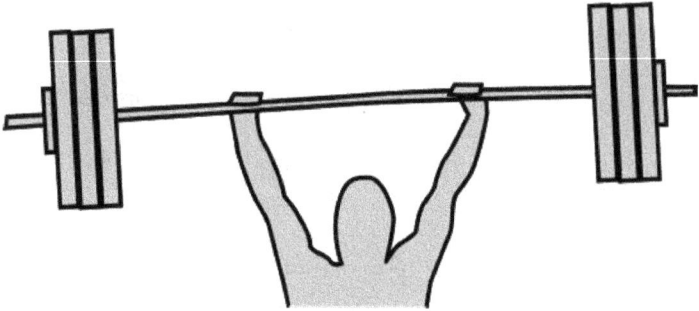

A. Hamstring stretching

The purpose of the exercise is to stretch the posterior muscles of the legs. This exercise can be done by lying on the floor or by using different stools or supports. Below, you can see the exercise performed by lying on the floor.

You may perform this exercise with the knee of the opposite leg to the elevated leg bent or straight, as seen in the pictures.

1. Lie on the floor.

2. Bend the knees and then extend one of your legs and lift it in the air.

3. Support it preferably from the area of the calf, as this way you stretch the back of the knee (not demonstrated in these pictures).

4. Keep this position for about 30-60 seconds (shorter time in the beginning) and control your breathing.

5. Repeat for 5-10 times (fewer initial stages).

6. Repeat the same with the other leg.

With knee bent

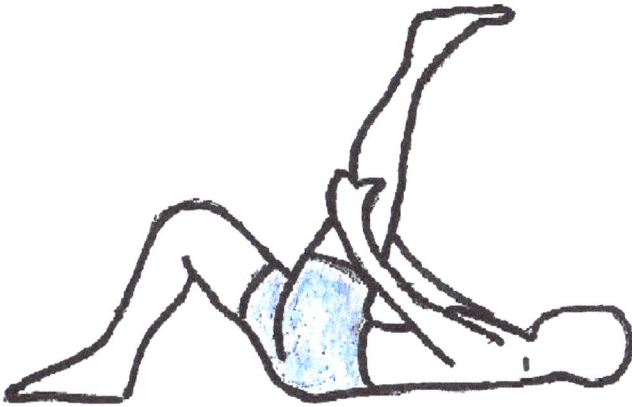

With knee straight

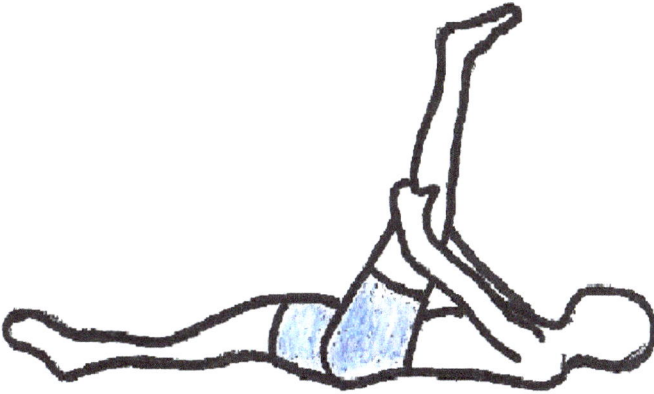

B. Pelvic tilt

1. Lie on your back (on the yoga mattress).

2. Bend your knees and keep your feet on the floor.

3. Make your abdominal (stomach) muscles tight.

4. Push your back against the floor.

5. Hold this position for 6-10 seconds, then increase the time to 10-30 seconds and relax.

6. Complete three sets of 10-15 repetitions.

The aim is to make isotonic contractions of the abdominal muscles, while also stretching the dorsal muscles of the spine at the same time. During this exercise, the iliopsoas muscle is also stretched.

Lying

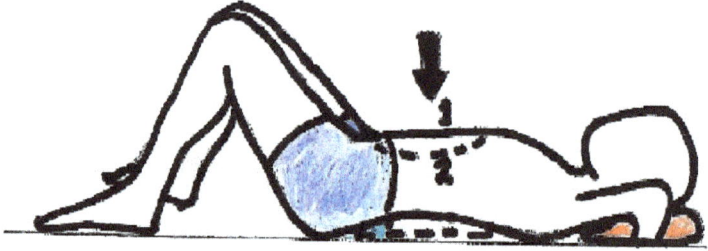

Standing

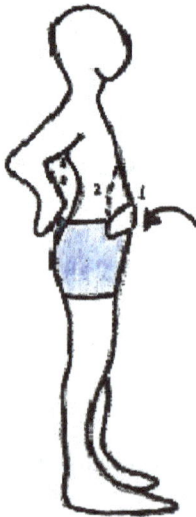

108

C. Partial curl

1. Stay on the floor lying on your back with knees bent and feet on the floor, as above.

2. Tighten your abdominal muscles.

3. Bend your neck, so your chin moves towards your chest.

4. Stretch your arms out in front of you.

5. Curl your upper body so your shoulders do not touch the floor.

6. Keep this position for 5-10 seconds and relax.

7. Complete 3 sets of 10-15 repetitions.

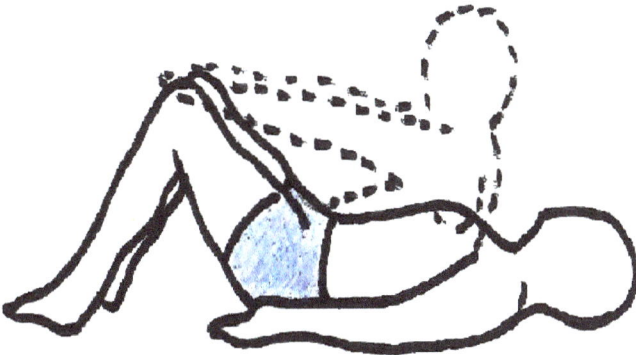

This is a strengthening exercise. The main active muscle is the rectus abdominis (six-pack muscle). The lateral abdominal muscles are also activated, albeit to a lesser degree.

With exercises like this, you stabilise your spine on the pelvis.

D. Gluteal stretch

1. Stay on the floor, lying on your back.

2. Keep one leg straight on the floor.

3. Bend the other knee towards your chest.

4. You will feel your gluteal (buttock) muscles stretching, as well as the muscles at the bottom of the spine and the back of the straight leg.

5. Hold this position for 20-60 seconds or for 5-10 breaths.

6. Repeat on the opposite side.

7. Complete three sets of 10-15 repetitions

The movements during this exercise should be gradual. During the initial stages, you may find that the range of movement at the hip joint is not full. Do not worry, as this will slowly improve.

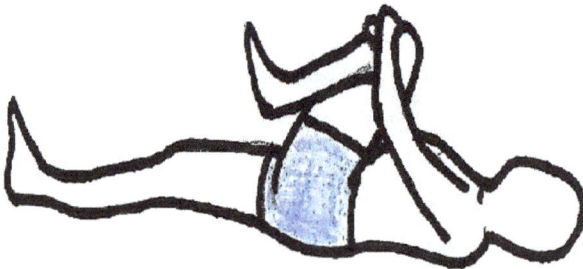

E. Modified/Alternative Gluteal stretch (Keep position for 10-30 seconds. Repeat 3-5 times per leg 10-20 times).

E1. Modified

1. Keep position as described in the previous section.

2. Flex the knee as before but add cross leg rotation.

3. As you hold this knee with your opposite hand, keep rotating and pushing it towards the floor on the opposite side.

4. Feel the stretching of the gluteal (buttock) and hip piriformis (lateral aspect rotator) muscles.

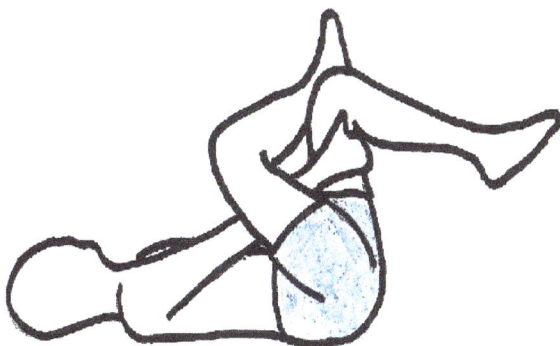

E2. Alternative

The same exercise can be done with the person facing down, kneeling on the floor. One leg should be straight on the floor and the other leg should be crossing straight under the body on the opposite side, with the knee flexed.

1. The arms should be extended straight forward as the person presses themselves down.

2. This exercise helps stretch the gluteal (buttock), piriformis

(lateral hip muscles), quadriceps (front thigh muscle), iliopsoas (muscle linking hip, pelvis, and spine), quadratus (dorsal muscle stabilising spine on pelvis), and lateral abdominal muscles on the extended leg.

3. Repeat the exercise with the other leg.

4. Hold for 5-10 breaths.

F. Stretching of lower back

1. Lie on your back.

2. Bend both legs at the hip joints.

3. Put your hands behind the knees.

4. Bend the knees.

5. Pull the thighs towards your chest and let the knees almost touch your face.

6. Feel the stretching of the lower back muscles.

7. Hold the position for 5-10 breaths.

8. Repeat 10-20 times.

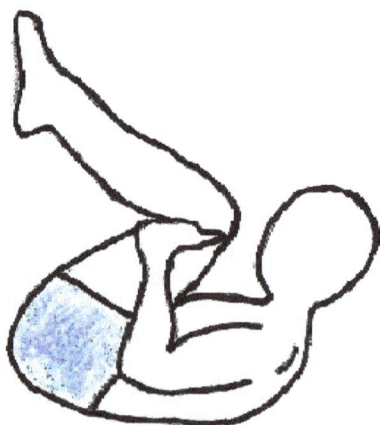

G. Stretching of lower back and lateral abdominal muscles

1. Lie down on your back.

2. Flex your hips and knees but keep your feet on the floor.

3. Extend your arms to the sides.

4. Rotate your knees either together to one side, trying to touch the floor with the side of the knee in the direction you are rotating (if the knees rotate towards the right, the lateral side of the right knee has to touch the floor), or one crossing over the other as you rotate the pelvis. During the exercise, concentrate on breathing, as you need to find a rhythm. Additionally, during exhalation, you may achieve more rotational movement. You can either keep the opposite arm to the rotation extended to stabilise yourself and achieve more muscle stretch, while the other could be under your head.

5. Feel the stretching in the lateral muscles of the lower back, as well as the lateral hip muscles.

6. Hold the position for 5-10 breaths.

7. Complete three to five sets of 10-20 repetitions.

8. Repeat the exercise for the opposite side.

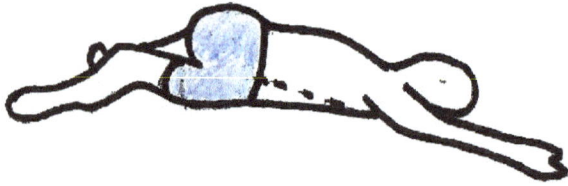

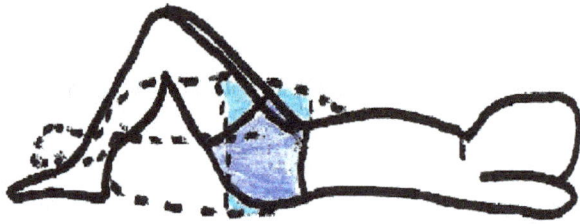

H. Double leg bridge

1. Keep lying on your back.

2. Knees your knees flexed, with your feet on the floor.

3. Keep your arm straight by the sides of your body.

4. Raise your pelvis from the ground towards the ceiling.

5. Hold for 10-15 seconds.

6. Repeat for 3-5 sets of 5-10 times.

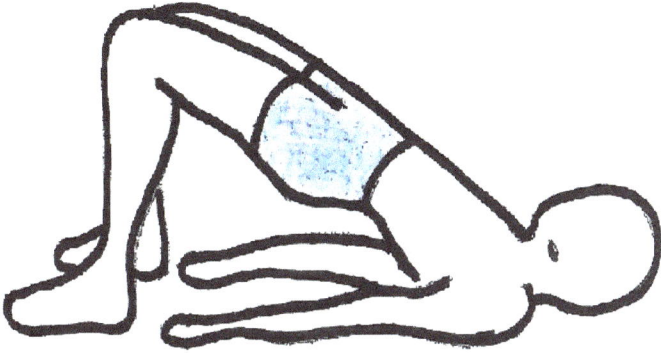

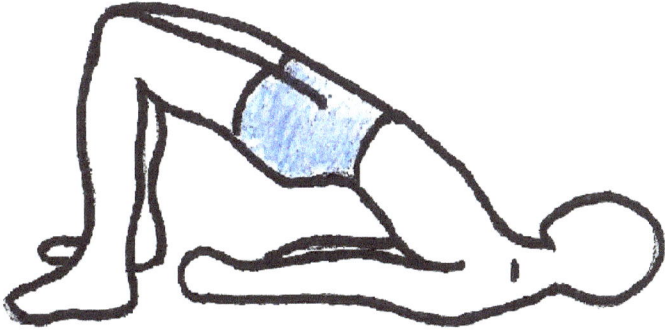

The aim of this exercise is to strengthen the core muscles (dorsal and abdominal) as well as the thigh muscles (quadriceps and hamstrings).

This is one of the final exercises that someone has to do.

I. Camel/Cat position
Cow

1. Get down on your hands and knees.

2. Relax your abdominal muscles and let your back "fall" towards the floor, creating a downward curvature.

3. Maintain this extended position for 10 seconds.

115

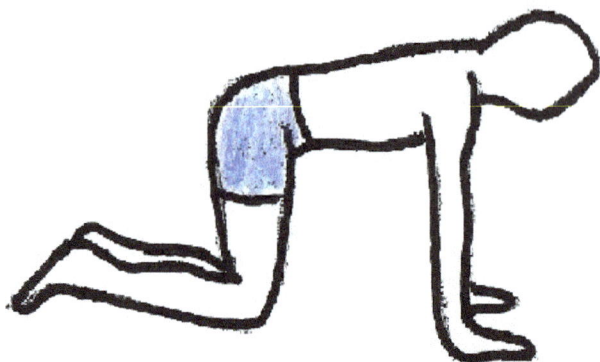

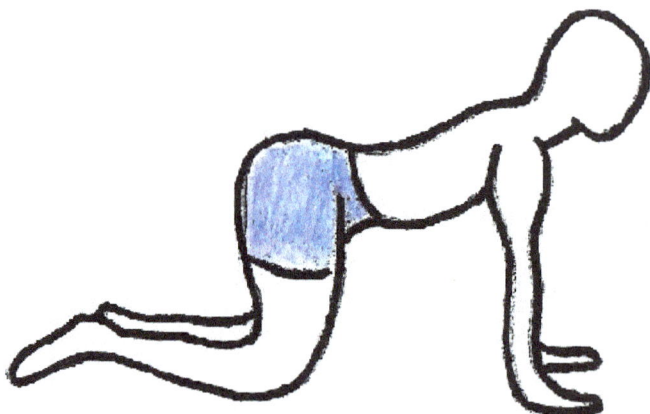

Cat/Camel

1. Tighten your abdominal muscles and arch your back upwards like a hump.

2. Hold this position for another 10 seconds.

3. Repeat 3-5 sets, of 10-20 times.

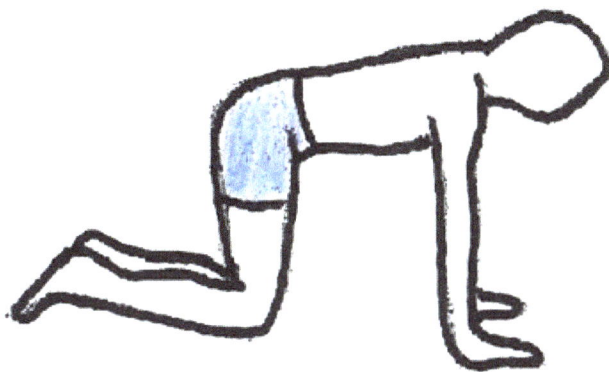

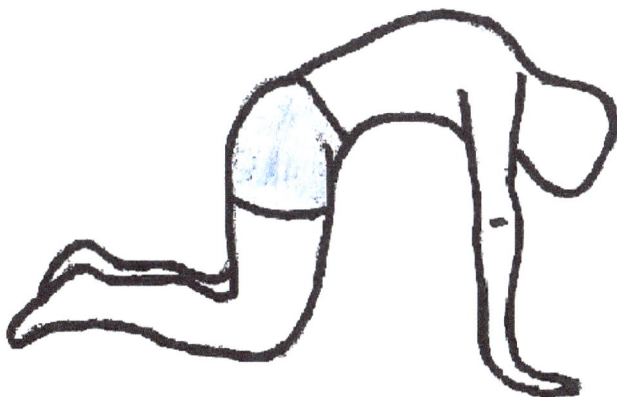

The combination of these exercises creates contractions as well as stretches to different muscle groups, depending on the position and which exercise is performed. The muscle groups involved are the abdominal and dorsal muscles, alternating between them.

Occasionally, it is possible for the muscles to develop cramps. In such cases, please relax and reverse the movement.

J. Quadruped – Half Superman

1. Stay down on your hands and knees.

2. Lift one arm and extend it forward overhead.

3. Then lift the opposite leg and extend it straight back.

4. Hold this position for 5-10 seconds.

5. Repeat on the opposite side.

6. Complete three sets of 10 repetitions.

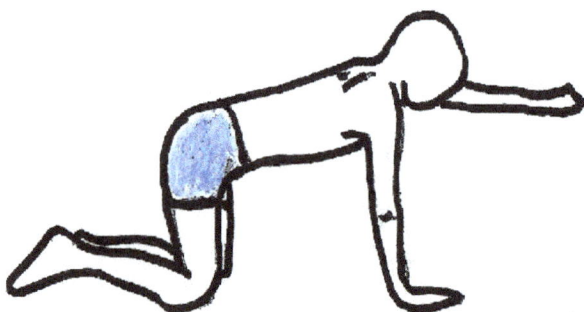

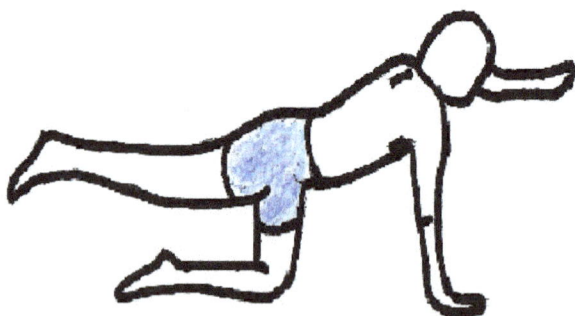

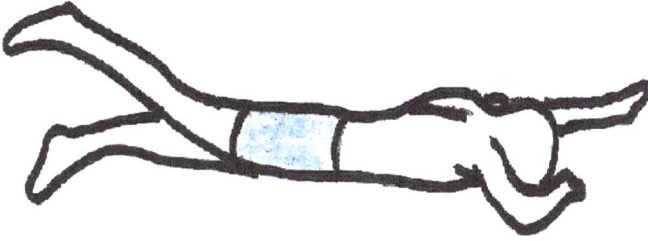

During these exercises, there is a combination of isometric and isotonic muscle contractions of several muscles. The main major muscles involved are the upper dorsal muscle, Trapezius, and at the lower body, the Glutei and Hamstrings.

K. Superman

1. Lie on your stomach.

2. Extend both arms forward overhead.

3. Extend the leg straight backwards.

4. Tighten the muscles of your back to lift part of your chest and your legs simultaneously off the floor.

5. Hold this position for up to 10 seconds.

6. Repeat for 3-5 sets, 10 repetitions.

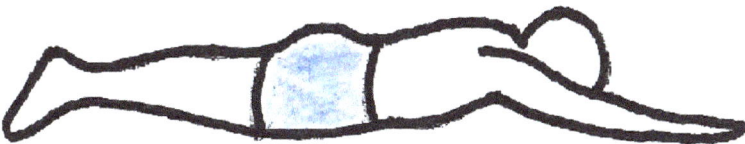

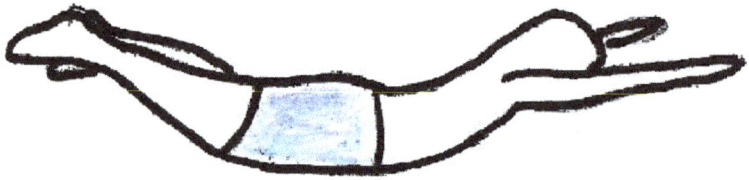

This is a strengthening exercise.

Isotonic exercises are a combination of different muscle groups, such as the dorsal muscles, the glutes, and hamstrings.

L. Turtle

1. Stay down on your hands and knees.

2. Flex your hips and knees as your bottom moves towards your feet.

3. Extend your arms straight overhead with the palms on the ground.

4. Your face comes close to the floor.

5. Stretch your body as if you are trying to reach something over your head, while pushing your hips away from your shoulders.

6. Feel the stretching of the back muscles.

7. Hold this position for 10 breaths.

8. Repeat for 3 sets of 10 times.

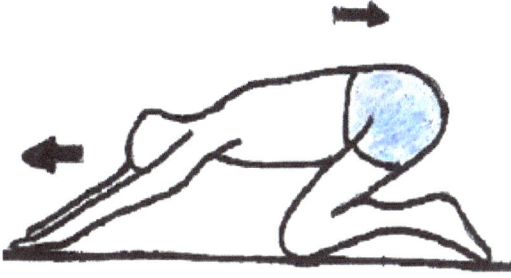

This is a stretching exercise that helps the muscles relax. Such an exercise can be done at the end of any session.

M. Cobra

1. Lie face down.

2. Place both hands at shoulder height.

3. Raise the upper torso from the ground as far as you can.

4. Keep the lower body relaxed.

5. Feel the squeeze of the dorsal muscles.

6. Stay in this position for 30 seconds or a minimum of 10 breaths.

7. Repeat 10 times.

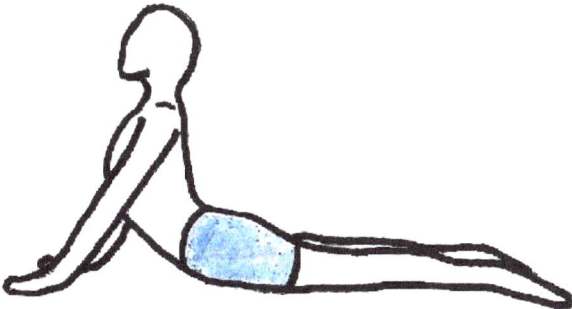

M1. Half cobra

- In case of difficulties extending at the initial stages, stabilise the upper body on the elbows instead of the hands.

- During this position, keep the angle between the elbow and forearm at 90 degrees, with the forearm extended forward.

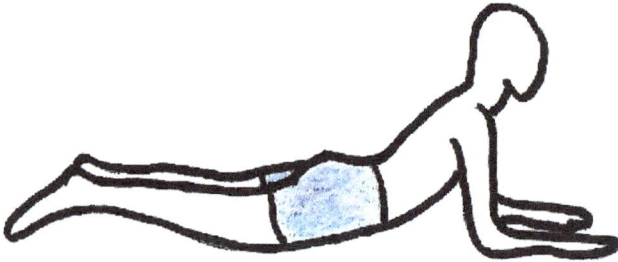

During these exercises, the back has to be relaxed, and the work has to be done by the arms and shoulders.

The purpose of this exercise is to potentially assist in gently repositioning a mildly posteriorly bulging disc, as the anterior intervertebral space opens up and may allow the nucleus to translate back into position.

Do not tense the muscles in the lower back at all.

N. Plank

1. Stay on the mattress facing down.

2. Place the elbows under your shoulders.

3. Extend the forearms on either side of your head.

4. Balance the upper body on the elbows, maintaining a 90-degree angle between the arm and forearm.

5. Tighten your dorsal/back muscles and lift your pelvis from the floor.

6. Keep the legs straight and balance on your toes.

7. Hold this position for 30 seconds and repeat 5-10 times, resting between repetitions.

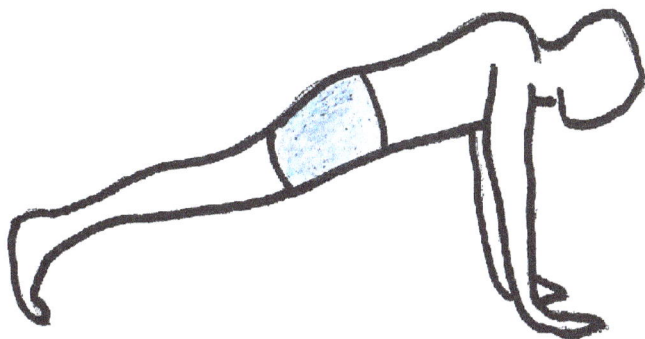

Static isometric exercises for strengthening the abdominal and dorsal muscles, as well as the iliopsoas, quadriceps, and glutei.

N1. Alternative plank

• If the described exercise is difficult to execute, instead of extending and balancing on toes, you can balance the lower part of your body on your knees.

• Progress to the plank position when your dorsal muscles become stronger.

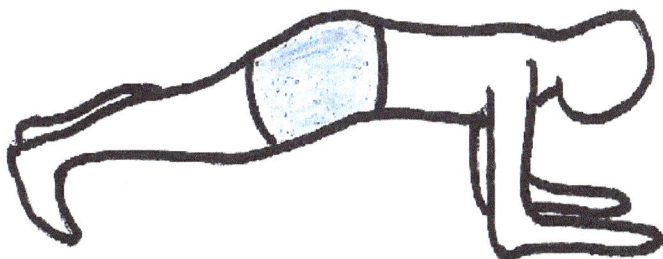

During these exercises, the dorsal muscles hold the pelvis in line, while the combined anterior and lateral abdominals contribute their strength and assist the dorsal muscles. The iliopsoas assists the thigh muscles, which collectively support the position of the upper leg and keep the knee locked in extension. The calf muscles are also involved in maintaining stability. In the upper part of the body, the trapezius is one of the main muscles that plays a role, with assistance from the other dorsal muscles.

O. Side plank

1. Lie on your side with your legs, knees, shoulders in a straight line.

2. Place your elbow under your shoulder and extend your forearm forward at a 90-degree angle.

3. Tighten your lateral abdominal muscles and lateral thigh muscles.

4. Raise your body (torso and pelvis) of the ground, balancing on your forearm-elbow complex on the top and lateral aspect of your foot at the bottom.

5. Hold this position for 30 seconds and repeat 5-10 times.

6. Rest between repetitions.

7. Repeat the same steps on the opposite side.

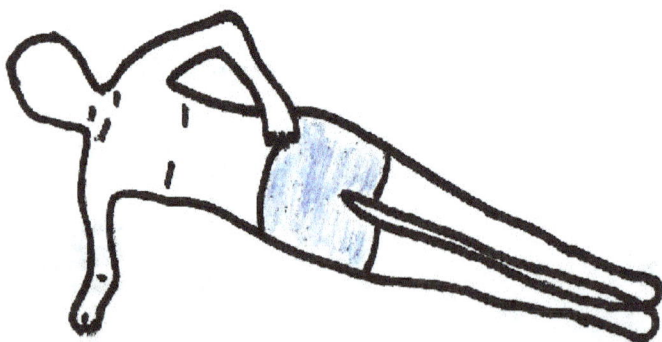

O1. Alternative side plank

Initially, if there is difficulty balancing the body on the elbow-forearm complex and feet, you can balance it on the elbow-forearm and lateral aspect of the knee.

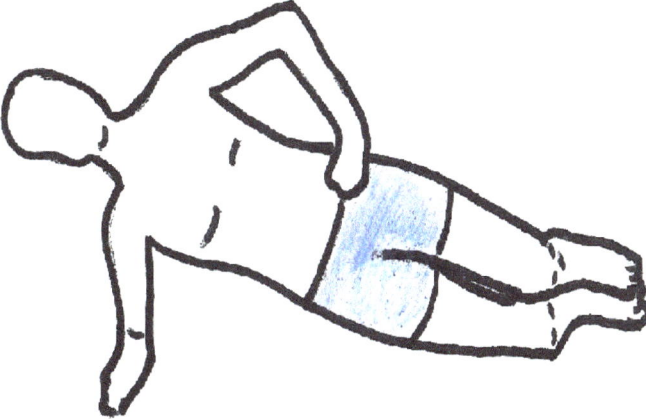

These are isometric exercises primarily involving the lateral abdominal muscles, although as described in the previous pages, other muscle groups are also engaged.

Start with a duration of 10 breaths.

P. Press ups

1. Face down on the mattress.

2. Place your hands under your shoulders.

3. Assume the plank position - arms straight, body off the floor.

4. Bend the arms at the elbow joint.

5. The body should be reaching the floor.

6. Push the body up again.

7. Complete three sets of 10 repetitions.

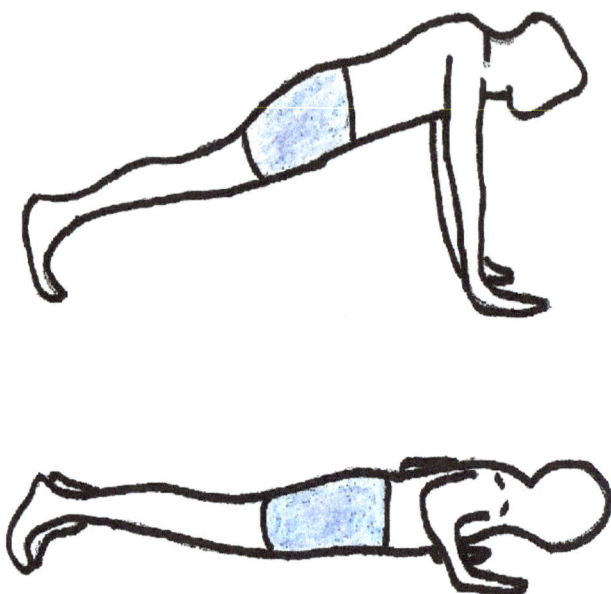

Active isotonic strengthening exercises for the pectoral and upper arm muscles (triceps and biceps), while simultaneously incorporating isometric exercises for the abdominal and dorsal muscles.

P1. Alternative Press ups

- Keep the alternative plank position.

- Repeat the elbow movements as explained above.

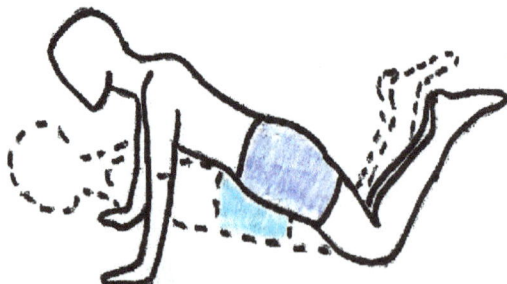

P2. Alternative Press up (version 2)

In case you have difficulty balancing your extended hands on the floor, you can use other objects instead (such as a wooden box, side of a bed, or a wall) and perform the same exercise.

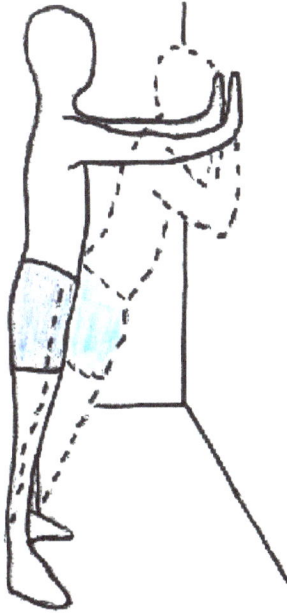

 These positions only help to reduce the load that goes through the upper body and facilitate you in case of difficulties performing proper press-ups.

Q. Rotational stretching of back in siting position

1.   Stay in a sitting position, on a chair or preferably on the floor. Keep one leg straight and bend the opposite leg, crossing it over the straight leg.

2.   Twist your body from one side back to a neutral position (neutral is when the face is looking forward).

3.   The torso pivots over the extended arm that is placed on the floor behind you, stabilising you.

4. The other arm is placed across the knee of the bent leg, and the elbow touches the knee.

5. Push with your knee against the arm, forcing torso rotation.

6. During this exercise, you stretch the lower back as well as the external rotator muscles of the hip.

7. Repeat the same on the opposite side.

8. Do three sets of 15-20 repetitions for each set.

9. You can repeat the exercise with the leg bent instead of straight.

10. You can repeat the exercise by placing your hands across your chest while remaining in a sitting position on the floor and do the same movements. However, there is no tension between the arms and knees.

11. During exhaling, you are stretching more as you try to rotate the body.

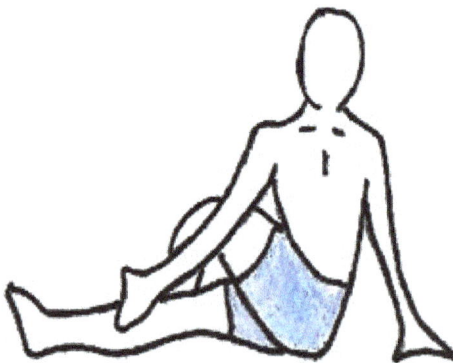

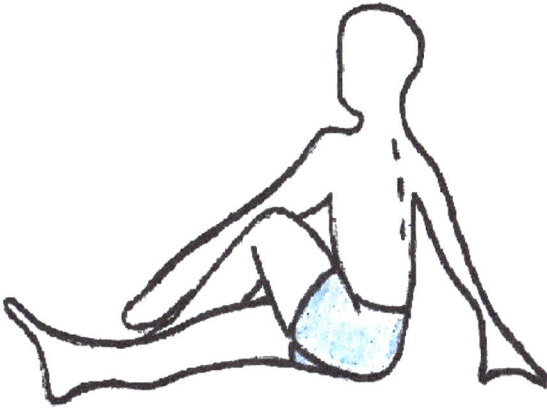

MEDITATION

I have a few options on this matter.

1. Taking long walks next to the ocean on the beach early in the morning, regardless of the weather conditions. Being close to the water and hearing the waves gives a great feeling of internal cleansing.

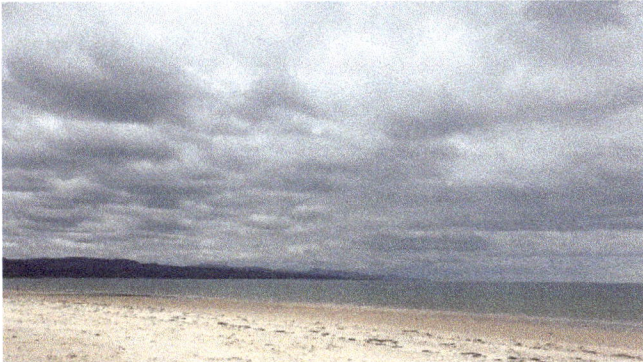

The sound of the waves and the rhythm of this sound are very comforting in the mind.

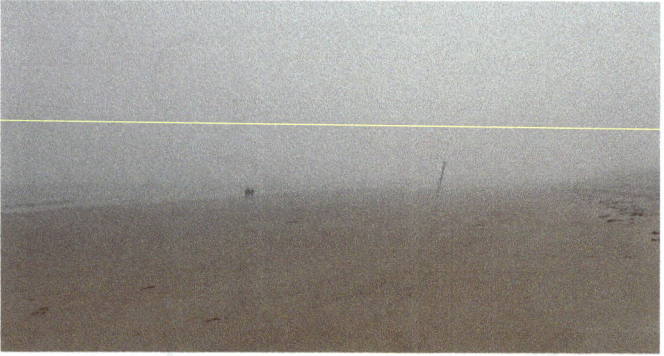

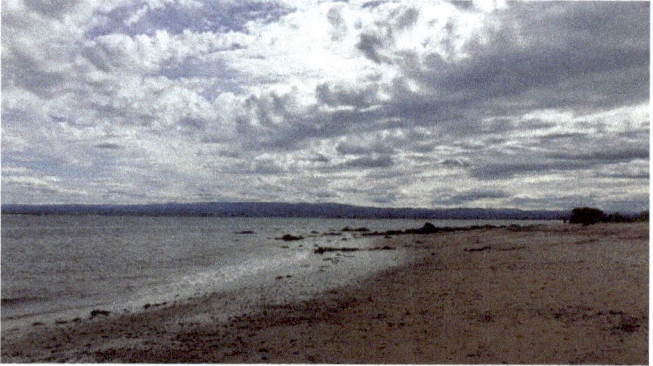

2. Sitting on a bench at the tip of the path on a small "cape" and spending hours next to the sea at that little spot at the end of the circular walking path. Admiring the natural beauty could be part of your "cure." The connection with the water is great.

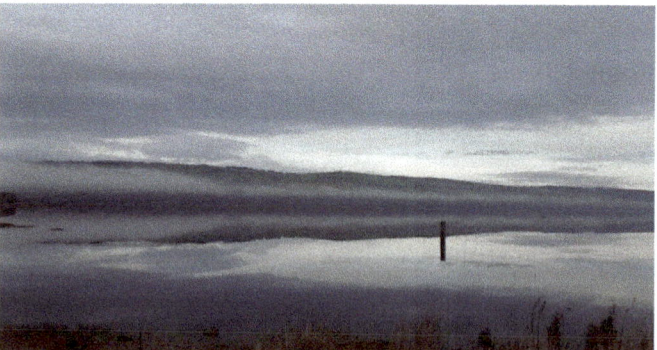

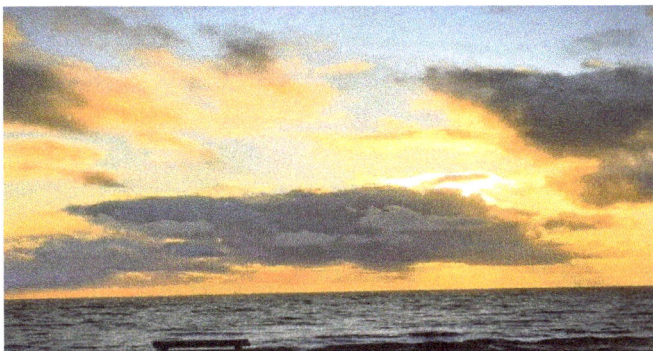

Nature has a great calming effect. Simply observing the reflection of mist on the still water in the distance evokes a feeling of admiration. How does Nature truly orchestrate such a scene? It is incredibly soothing.

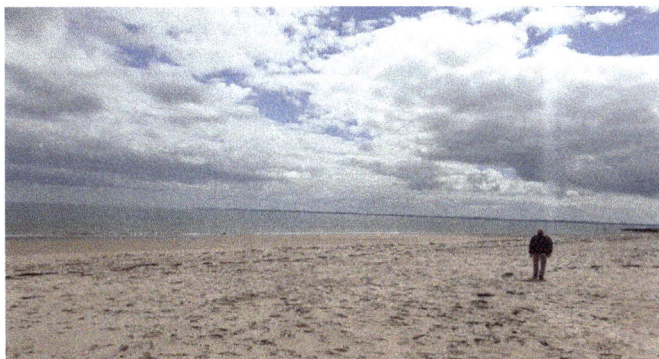

3. A walk through the forest next to a river with waterfalls. The sound of the falling water is great, as it is the sound of nature calling you to be energised.

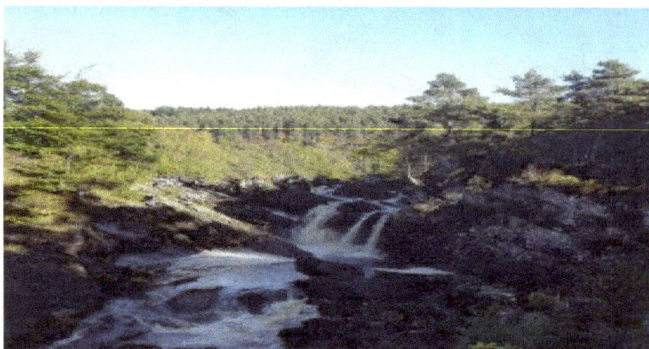

The running water takes away all the negative thoughts you have and flows them down to the sea.

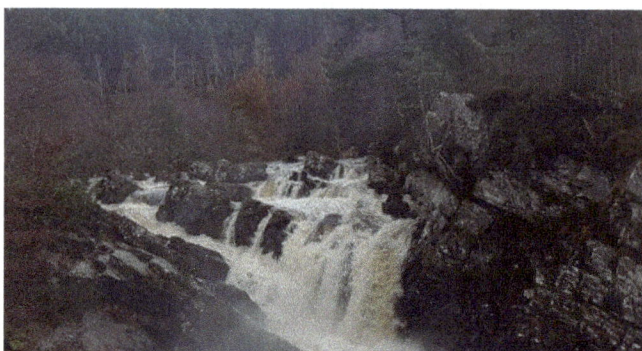

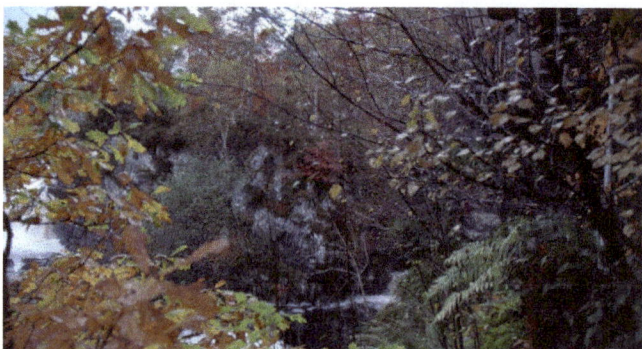

BREATHING EXERCISES

Under soft music, you can perform breathing exercises, focusing inward and finding pleasurable thoughts about your life.

MENTAL AWARENESS

To achieve this, you may need several tools, such as changing your mindset, beliefs, and habits. It is proven to be the most difficult part of life.

You can start by answering the following fundamental questions:

1. Where are you?

2. Where do you want to go?

3. Why do you need to do this?

4. What do you have to do to achieve change?

5. How will you do it?

Where are you?
This is the starting point. Accept your condition; you have back pain. You cannot deny it, but you can confront it. It all starts here. You need to answer honestly. Reflect on the depth of your mind and confirm that this is point zero. You cannot achieve any goals if you don't know what your present circumstances are. Accept the realities of your life, let go of the judgmental view you have of yourself, and make the effort to begin the change. Be honest about your present situation. Remove any signs of self-pity and accept yourself as you are. If you don't know the starting point of your path at the beginning of your walk, you will not be able to map it.

How can you find it, though? There are the following reasons for you to be here at this moment. You either want to avoid pain, or you have to find a happy result in your life, or I believe both. Possibly, your back pain is not treated up to your satisfaction, either due to the proposed treatment itself or the deep understanding about the condition, or you have not found yet the way to entertain your back pain and make a happy compromise with it so you can live a more pleasurable life.

So stop and think where you are now. What is your current situation? What are your physical symptoms? How do they influence your emotional world? How does your family or broad social environment react? What is your behaviour towards yourself or the people around you? What is your connection with the Higher Power? The most important question, though, is: what is your opinion about yourself?

Answer honestly, but also think that you are still alive, and you are blessed to be able to react and change your life for the better. These positive thoughts have to guide you; concentrate on them but also analyse any negative feelings, as you have to be aware of what you really need to replace with positivity. You need the energy to start and launch the beginning of your journey as the fuel and energy that are necessary for the launch of a rocket at Cape Canaveral. The rocket consumes and burns tons of fuel to achieve a lift-off, starting the amazing journey. But all starts at Cape Canaveral. Find yours.

Write down your thoughts and feelings (mental and physical).

Where do you want to go?

What is your destination? In six months or a year from now, what do you think you want to achieve? What is the life you want to have? What connection do you want to have with your partner? Possibly, this is the most difficult question someone would ask you to answer. The majority of people know the problems they have and can list them in detail, but they never analyse their destination. Possibly, they imagine a place without the presence of these specific problems. I use the word "analyse" because they are living with this day-to-day problem and are used to firefighting, forgetting that by creating a strategic plan, they may resolve the issue. This is the reason they don't think about their future goals. If someone has to resolve any issues, they need to know the end result and the end destination. You have to imagine your end result and create a path that you have to follow. Think of this destination as a lighthouse in the distance and try to go there. Be smart and avoid the rocks, though.

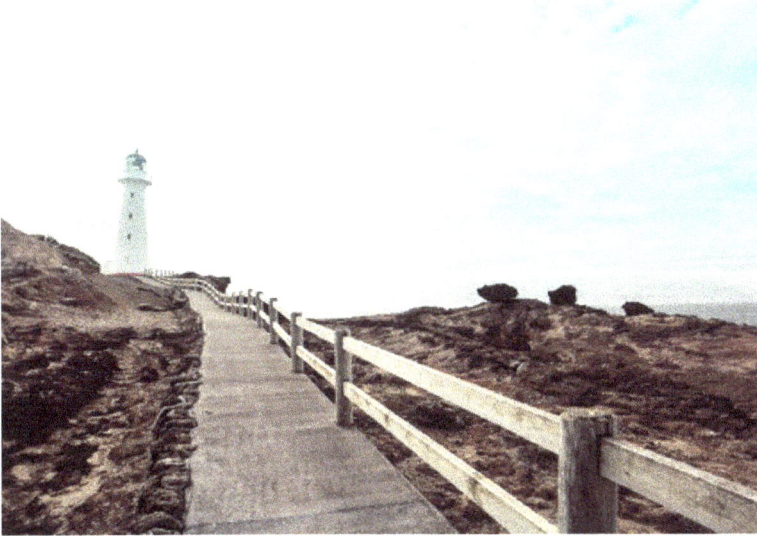

All of us remember the poster of the man who, using his index finger, pointed at each of us and asked us to do something. During the Second World War, as we see in films, his words were "Your country needs you." Nowadays, he is asking us to donate blood or organs. This demonstrates the power of the index finger. We follow it.

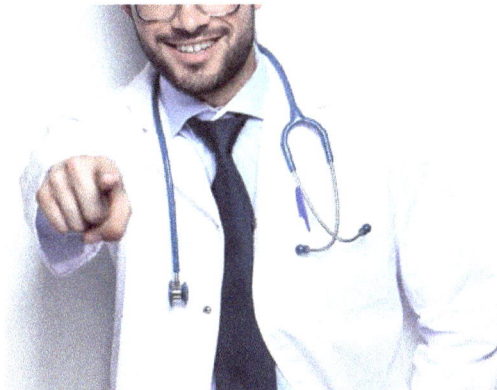

Concentrate on positive thoughts and follow them. It is not easy or comfortable. You have to take uncomfortable action and go for it. If you want to build six-pack muscles, photoshop one of your pictures where the six packs are evident and pin it on the fridge to see it every day. The same goes if you want to change your BMI. But on this picture, add some emotional thought. It is pointless to pin the picture and see it with an empty mind or think as you pass in front of the fridge, "I will be like this." You have to see the picture and vividly think, "I will look like Hercules, strong and healthy, and to do this I have to exercise because this is my goal."

Focus on this future image, destination, or goal. Pretend that you are there, six or twelve months from now, and you are celebrating your achievement. During this party, someone comes up to you and asks how you have done it. To answer this, you have to look back, follow the steps you walked from the start, and explain all this to that person. You know the steps. You have to be fluent. Describe all the way to your goal using colours with passion and be alive. Do not describe the story in black, grey, and white.

Now that you know the path, sit down, and write what goal you really want to achieve, what will be your destination, and pretend you are there. Write down that you may want to live a life without pain or that you want six-pack abs, or that you have achieved a normal BMI, and now turn back and see the path you walked, all the steps taken, visualise every step, and write down how you achieved it.

Make a realistic plan. You have to achieve it but celebrate every single step of your achievement. This plan has to be down-to-earth. You will be neither anxious nor depressed if you set unrealistic goals and are unable to fulfil them. If your goal is to lose 20kg of weight in seven days, which is a fantasy, but you manage to lose 5kg, don't be unhappy. Your initial expectations were unrealistic but celebrate the positive step you took towards your long-term goal of weight loss.

But all this you have to write, make it vivid. Do not write the path, your plan, and your achievements in a bullet point list. Write it all with "colour."

If you wanted more money, for example, you would not write "I want money in the bank account" or "I want this expensive car," but you will imagine yourself within the car, going to the beach, and enjoying the sunshine with the roof down. This is the emotional picture. Create pictures. I hope it is clear. On the other hand, as the plan is to manage back pain, if you want to control your weight and visualise yourself with fewer kilos than before, elaborate on the picture. Write about your athletic, slim body. Write about the pleasure you will feel when you are in your swimsuit. Write about the long, intimate, loving moments you will spend with your significant other on a tropical island. Close your eyes and see the picture within your mind. Create an ideal movie of your future life. You need to add emotion. Emotion helps our imagination.

Why do you need to do this?

This is another question you have to think deeply about. Why do you want to change? Is it because you don't want to be in pain? Is that the only reason, or is it because the quality of your life is in ruins, and you want to make it better? Have you lost your job and want to find a new one but cannot? Do you have problems with your partner and are upset about it? Is it because you have put on a lot of weight and want to lose it?

If any of the above is the reason, you have to find out the answers. But if you have a different goal, then find out the answer to a different question. As soon as you find that this is your purpose, you have to ask yourself, do you have the energy to propel yourself toward this goal?

To answer all of this, you have to reflect within your soul and answer a series of questions that may feel repetitive, although this is not entirely true. Grammatically, it is the same question, but the meaning of it is different every time as it drives you deeper and deeper into your thoughts. Every question is based on the answer you give to the previous one. This was proposed and developed by my tutor and mentor, Dean Graziosi, who is an author, educator, founder of self-development, and a great believer in the changes education can achieve for all of us.

It is called the 7 Levels Deep and the questions are:

1. What is important to you, knowing what back pain is?

2. Why is important to you?

3. Why is important to you?

4. Why is important to you?

5. Why is important to you?

6. Why is important to you?

7. Why is important to you?

In every step, you have to ask "Why" based on the previous answer. So, this is what I mean by saying that the questions have a different meaning, although grammatically are the same.

You can also use a well-known tool for reflection, the De Bono, Six Thinking Hats tool. The hats represent different perspectives: White hat for gathering facts, Red hat for analysing emotions, Green hat for focusing on creativity, possibilities, and new ideas, Yellow hat for exploring the positive aspects and symbolising optimism, Black hat for symbolising caution and critical thinking in analysing problems (do not overuse it), and Blue hat for focusing on how the situation is or should be managed. However, the 7 Levels Deep technique may give you a better understanding and created an emotional anchor to your reasoning.

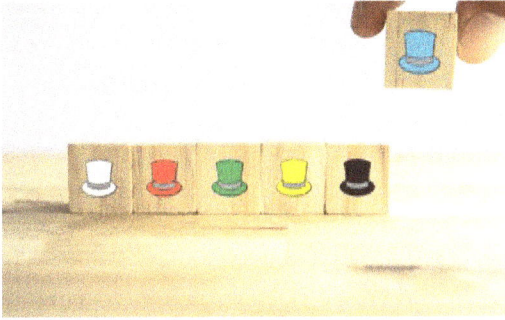

You need to find out why. By finding it, you will amplify your desire for the change you want. You have to write it down and implant it within your brain. It is known that if you do this, you will find that the focus point is getting closer and bigger.

Let us use potential answers as examples to answer the 7 Level Deep questions:

1. What is important to you, knowing what back pain is?

I want to come out of this daily torture of pain, and I want to know what is causing it.

2. Why is important to you come out of the daily torture?

I cannot live with the morning stiff back, and I want to be relaxed and happy.

3. Why is important to you to stop the morning stiff back and how will you be relaxed?

Every morning, it takes time for me to get out of bed and I need to take painkillers to improve my movement. I am unsteady and I need to support myself on the furniture until I will be able to slowly improve my posture. This is creating a lot of anxiety. I do not know how long this will take and I am not a happy person.

4. Why is important for you to become a happy person?

139

Because these mood swings affect my whole life. At work, I am moody, and I don't know if there will be a moment when I will speak in a different tone to any of the patients. I lost my patience, and this is dangerous.

5. Why is important to you to get your patience back?

To effectively serve people, I need to have patience and actively listen to them and their problems, with an aim to solve them. Without patience, I will be unable to assist anyone, and it will reflect negatively on my character. Additionally, it is crucial for me to be able to manage my emotions.

6. Why is important to you to control your emotions?

My emotions influence my behaviour, and this is affecting my family life. My spouse is getting agitated as when she is trying to help me, I fear that she will do something wrong. I am trying to push her away. My behaviour makes me angry.

7. Why is important to you to stop being angry?

Because this affects my overall well-being, I would like to live in a calm, positive, and non-traumatic environment. However, I cannot do so, and this may cause problems in my future life and lead to losing the love of my life. I want to be healthy, happy, safe, and confident in order to have a successful family life and bring my partner back.

After reviewing these responses, I may have answered some of your questions. Please take a moment to honestly reflect and answer the 7 'Why' questions in your own words.

What do you have to do to achieve change?

What are the tools or powers that you need to help you move forward and achieve your goals?

In my opinion, all these tools are within your reach. You already have them. You have your body, your own body, and your mind, your own mind. You are now able to understand how the body interacts with the mind and how you can use this knowledge to manipulate it in a way that allows you to achieve your goals. You need to take uncomfortable actions, change your beliefs, convince yourself that you can do it, and step out of your comfort zone to start taking action.

If you want positive change in your current circumstances, you need to give up the attitude of defending them. You must be willing to change. Willingness is a state that allows you to engage with your life and see situations from a new perspective.

"Where the willingness is great, the difficulties cannot be great" - Niccolo Machiavelli.

It requires focus, concentration, perseverance, determination, and self-assurance. By changing your beliefs, you unlock enormous potential within your physical and mental reserves. With action, you will be able to change the results to the level you desire. This may be a long process, and it will definitely take you out of your comfort zone and require a lot of work. It will not happen overnight.

Do not be afraid of failure. Embrace the paradox of seeing failure as a win. There are two perspectives on this argument. Failure is a win because subconsciously, you may have planned for it from the beginning. You may have never truly believed that your plan would be successful. It is similar to a failed marriage. You may have subconsciously thought that you were not worthy of a successful relationship, possibly due to past experiences. So, in a way, you successfully "won" your failure because you had planned for it all along without even realising it. On the other hand, failure can also be a win because it represents a lesson that you can learn from and avoid repeating. With all this in mind, do not fear failure, but be positive and avoid it by using a well-planned strategy.

You may ask, though, if we can be certain of the future success of our actions.

Here lies another paradox, the paradox of certainty. I would argue that it is not possible to be certain of any success. If we do not venture beyond the surface of uncertainty and step out of our routine comfort zones, we will not improve our current circumstances, and that is certain. Chasing certainty is essentially chasing something that does not exist because nothing in life is certain except for the future demise of each one of us. So, if nothing is certain, we can say that everything is uncertain. Why, then, do we fear uncertainty when we already live within it? It is the false feeling of comfort that numbs our minds. It is fear. So, stop fearing uncertainty and embrace it. Only then will you see change.

But you may say to me that you have thoughts that everything will remain as it is, that nothing will change, and that everything will fail. These are negative thoughts. Do you have negative thoughts? Do not fear them. Everyone has them. They are a part of our primitive brain. Do not let them define you. You are defined by your actions, not your thoughts. Those around you see your actions, and no one knows your thoughts. Separate your thoughts from your actions. Act in a positive and assertive way, even if your brain fills you with negativity. Negativity will keep coming if you allow it to through inactivity. Fight back; persist in a routine that pushes away any negative thoughts. Take positive action. This is the only solution. Action builds your confidence, and confidence helps you overcome any negativity. Be in control of yourself and your life. This is freedom.

"A man who cannot control self is not free" - Pythagoras.

How will you do it?

What do you think you will need to have in order to achieve your goals?

Dr. Daniel Amen, renowned neuropsychologist, has said in his teachings that you have to love your brain and support it. You have to provide it with the correct nutrition. Nutrition for the brain represents not only the correct substances that will arrive there through the blood supply, but also the correct thoughts. He uses a nice terminology that creates a vivid picture. He says that you have to protect your brain from ANTs (Autonomous Negative Thoughts), as these can erode your brain.

He states that everyone needs to have positive thoughts and keep their brain happy.

Everyone knows what will make them unhappy. Try to reflect and find out the reasons for your unhappiness, write them down, and make it your goal to avoid them.

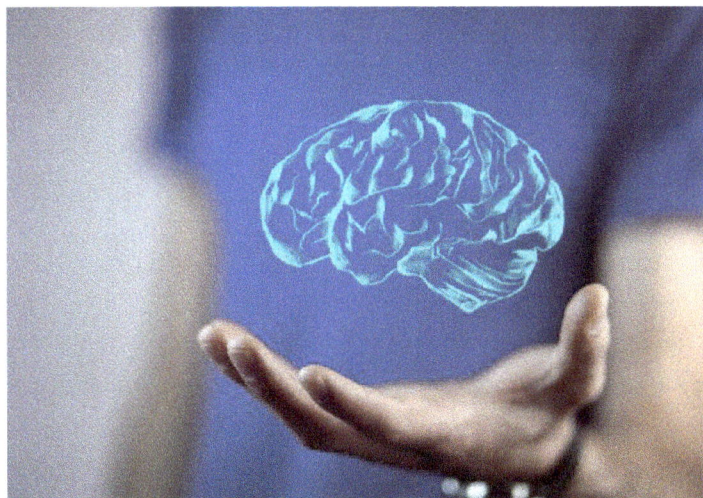

Sit down and write down all the unhappy moments and what created these feelings, whether mental or physical, and consciously start to avoid them. Possibly, the physical ones could be easier to detect, while the mental ones may come to the surface much later.

Use the tools available to overcome anxiety and physical symptoms. As I mentioned before, try using the 7-level deep technique or the 6 thinking hats. Use them to try and find a path for action.

In other words, try to understand your body better. To achieve this, you have to change your mindset. Change your habits and in turn, change your life, and you will become happier.

Reflect on yourself, take uncomfortable action, and achieve a life free from a sedentary lifestyle filled with fear and disappointment. Instead, lead an active life where you manage the results and improve your pain. Change more than just your back pain. Change your overall health. Change your perspective about back pain and stop panicking when it occurs. The solution is in your hands. Enjoy your love life.

In this printed material, you have all the information that will help you understand how the spine functions and how you can improve your symptoms. It contains everything you need if you want to start your journey towards a better life without pain. You need to find the ways to implement what is possible for you, so you can bring about the desired change. Please, I urge you to take action.

MARKING DOWN

Exercises can help you control your BMI (Body Mass Index). To improve, follow some rules. Experiment by using healthy diets until you find the one that works and makes you happy. A sensible way is to replace a lot of your meals with vegetables and salads. At the same time, take the desirable amount of proteins throughout the day by adding either fish or lean poultry to your diet. Red meat could be consumed rarely, but don't remove it completely. Sodas must be completely removed, but alcohol, only red wine, salt, and sweets could be consumed very rarely. Look after your gut.

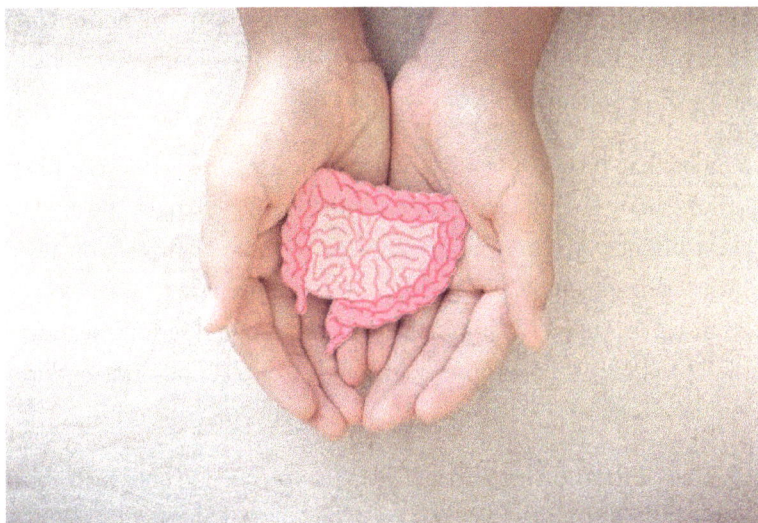

In addition, intermittent fasting could be added if you wish to. The first ten (10) days of fasting application may be very difficult. To combat hunger, keep busy and try to avoid giving in to your cravings. You can initially implement a 16:8 fasting schedule (16 hours of fasting and 8 hours to eat). Be careful not to overeat during the 8-hour eating window. It is not helpful at all. Alternatively, you could follow a 2:5 schedule (fast for two days out of five) and complement this with your exercise routine.

Hippocrates, the father of Medicine, said that *"Let food be the medicine and medicine be the food."*

This is true. You need to follow the rules and have a balanced intake of a diversity of nutritious foods that will be beneficial to your body.

In addition, keep your microbiome happy and your body rejuvenated by using autophagy.

But really, if you ask me, I don't think that only the diet itself makes the difference. You need discipline to count your calories and make sure that you will not go over the amount calculated for you.

There are applications you can load to your phone too. Start adding everything you are eating in that. The application will automatically calculate your calories and by adding everything, you could avoid cheating. This way, you could control your weight.

Remember that BMI control is a journey in itself, based on the physical changes the body goes through as well as the mental changes you are forced to have without your knowledge. To reverse these changes, you need to transform yourself physically and mentally and prepare yourself to accept that to travel from A to Z, it may be difficult in one nonstop journey. You may need to accept that stopping in K for a bit is good and re-planning may be necessary.

You need to be transformed. To achieve this, you need to believe in yourself and change. You need to have integrity, meaning that you will follow and make reality the plan you created at the timescale you said it will happen. This is linked directly with your self-respect and self-discipline. To achieve your goal, you need to plan to walk in small achievable steps and this will help your confidence. Being confident will help your ability to change your beliefs as you realistically see the difference. Do not lose faith in case of delays within your journey and have a person near you who may help your journey. Humans are social "animals." A friend will hold your hand and assist you in the journey, pointing out your achievements and not the failures. Be positive.

In summary, the elements you need to conclude your journey are integrity, dignity, discipline, dedication to detail, perseverance, focus, inner light, patience, becoming part of a positive helpful community, and most of all honesty. Be honest with yourself and others. Have your values and act according to them.

Finally, I am not going to suggest any of these schemes, whether it be diet or fasting patterns, directly to you, as what worked for me may not work for you. This material is for educational purposes only. Please consider what you believe is relevant to you. Base your decisions on your own cultural and intellectual

background and accept only what aligns with it. Discover what works for you through experimentation and consult your personal physician for further advice.

Activity

Write down what you need to avoid and make it a goal to eliminate them from your life.

_____

_____

_____

Choose the exercises that you are able to do.

Find your own ways to meditate.

Design your diet with or without the help of a physician, but remain dedicated to the instructions and measure everything.

Answer the 7 level deep questions again and again.

EPILOGUE

Let us start with the analysis of life as Epicurus, the Greek philosopher, saw it and taught about it so many centuries ago. His main teaching was based on these four sentences that he called Tetrapharmakos (the four-part cure).

1. Don't fear God.

2. Don't worry about death.

3. What is good is easy to get.

4. What is terrible is easy to endure.

I am talking about the analysis of these doctrines but allow me to only focus on the last two, as the others do not touch on the subject of the book as obviously.

Starting with the last one, the man is saying that anything bad and ugly that comes and hits us is "welcomed," as we have the physical and mental abilities to overcome it. And in the case of this book, which deals with back pain, it is clear that the "terrible" encounter for your miserable body is this burden; the back pain, and mainly the chronic one, which tortures you physically and mentally.

Additionally, this back pain is destroying your life. You are unable to function. It is not possible to move without noticing it. Your body is changing shape as your chemistry is derailed and there is a whole lot of hormonal imbalance. Fear, stress, anxiety, and desperation are controlling your life and filling all the space around you. You are unable to breathe freely. You are getting depressed, retreating to the dark side of your inner existence like traumatised animals, searching for the cure that only time provides to all. You have lost your motivation and confidence for life and deny yourself anything that drives you to a life of pleasure. In case someone around you feels a glimpse of joy, anger, and envy are filling your mind.

But what did he say?

He said that you are able to endure and overcome the "terrible."

But how, you may ask?

It is time to see what he is telling you above the last quote.

What is good is easy to get.

But what is good?

Good is everything that reverses your misery. Good is the smile of your loved ones. Good is the sunlight. Good is the shining moon. Good is the breeze that comes from the sea or the sound of running water or the tweeting of birds.

You notice that good is all around you. It is provided to you by nature. Good is nature.

What can be more natural than existing with your partner, embraced and hugging, living that special moment of absolute connection?

The means to battle against back pain are within your reach. Mobility, music, aromatic smells, special tasteful foods, or beautiful pictures are able to fill your lives and change the course of your mental understanding. You have to use all your senses and build up your sensuality. You can fight back pain and live a happy, full life - a life where pleasure exists and pain will stop robbing this from you.

The only thing you need to do is believe in your abilities, find ways and be resourceful, but most importantly, you must not lose your motivation for progress and have the ability to take action that could build up your confidence. Confidence is your defence mechanism for anything that hits you directly.

Communication, care, respect, love, gentle touch, the taste of a lover's kiss are something that can clear the mist of pain and bring pleasure back into the previously thought-to-be-painful life. It is called sex therapy, mainly focusing on motion, but this is not the only improvement you may have from such activities.

These actions bring hormonal balance back to better levels, improve pain, and help you become motivated, confident, and reassured that your life is great again.

You must not stop believing that you can have intimacy back in your life. We have to abandon thoughts of guilt and despair. Life is beautiful and you have, all of you have to live it in full, selflessly, supporting each other, and believing in your own powers.

For all of you, please apply the Epicurean Tetrapharmakos (four-part cure) and mainly the third and fourth parts of it: "What is good is easy to get and What is terrible is easy to endure." Epicurus (Greek philosopher) believed that "Continuous pain does not last long, even if it is extreme, it will be present only for a short period and you have the ability to overcome it, if you can recognise the physical and mental limits and you can endure it, if you can become confident that there is pleasure only to follow the pain and nothing else."

Focus on these words, but most of all, his master quote: "Find your tranquillity."

Reading all this, you will find that avoidance of intimacy is based on fear, something you have to abolish. Inability to perform sexual acts is a myth. You need to communicate your fears, limitations, educate yourself, and trust your significant other. You both are a team. You can find solutions to the issues you have, as these are common for both of you.

Do all activities with care, love, respect, and after communication. You can do this.

Do not allow pain to rob you of pleasure.

Activity

> Reflect and write down a journal of all thoughts applying to the 5 P's, 5 M's, and do the 7 Levels Deep.

> Reflect to find the reasons why your back pain is getting worse.

> Become aware of your daily habits and thoughts that are linked to your back pain. Eliminate negative thoughts and replace them with positive actions.

> Plan your ideal future and work towards it, one step at a time.

> Apply the exercises and increase your movement.

> Move away from your sofa.

Plan the first task you have to do and concentrate on it. Once you are content and focused, plan the diversion to give attention to a second task. Do not become obsessed with only one goal. Check your ability to achieve the goals separately by taking one step at a time. Plan the steps to achieve your final goal.

Change your attitude towards mechanical low back pain; initially, it is your friend, and if you think it becomes your enemy, try to go back to having a friendly relationship with it. Do not fight it, but "negotiate" with it.

Communicate with your loved ones, trust them, explain limitations, and believe in your abilities.

Be sensual and do not let the pain rob you of your pleasure.

Remember

Back pain is a symptom.

Please do not allow it to become a syndrome.

IMPORTANT NOTICES / DISCLAIMERS

The depicted experience may not be considered as typical. Your background, education, experience, and work ethic may differ. This is used as an example and not a guarantee of success. Individuals do not track the typicality of its student's experiences. Your results may vary.

The contents of this training, such as text, graphics, images, and other material are intended for informational and educational purposes and not for the purpose of rendering medical or mental health advice. The contents of this training are not intended to substitute for professional medical advice, diagnosis, and/or treatment. Please consult your medical professional before making changes to your diet, exercise routine, medical regimen, lifestyle, and/or mental health care.

This is not a medical consultation or medical advice. This is a guide to be followed, aiming to improve the quality of your life. You can keep all material necessary to you and discard what is not working for you.

Stories shared during the sessions of the modules are true experiences of me personally, or of patients that have crossed paths with me during consultations many years ago. No personal details are shared within the course that can make them identifiable to anybody.

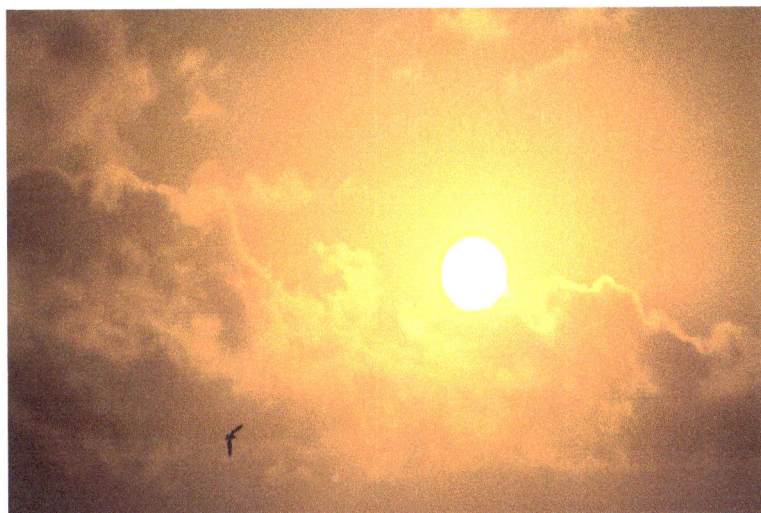

Follow the Light

EVALUATION

I would be grateful if you could take the time to complete the following questionnaire and email it to faceyourbackpain1@gmail.com:

1. Please tick the correct grading on the table, (1 for the least relevant and 5 for the most relevant to you)

Statements	1	2	3	4	5
Was the content something you were expecting?					
Was the given information easy to understand?					
Were the illustrations clear?					
Did this material improve your knowledge?					
Was the material useful to you?					
Do you feel better after this?					

2. Please write below on what we can do better

_____

_____

_____

_____

_____

_____

3. Please answer the following questions:

- What were you like before the course?

_____

_____

_____

- How did the course made you feel?

_____

_____

_____

- What did you like most about it?

_____

_____

_____

- What changes have you made, following the course?

_____

_____

_____

Thank you very much for allowing me to share my experience with you and serve you.

Thank you